INDIGENOUS HEALTH
AND JUSTICE

Indigenous Justice

MARIANNE O. NIELSEN AND KAREN JARRATT-SNIDER
Series Editors

INDIGENOUS HEALTH AND JUSTICE

EDITED BY
KAREN JARRATT-SNIDER AND
MARIANNE O. NIELSEN

THE UNIVERSITY OF
ARIZONA PRESS
TUCSON

The University of Arizona Press
www.uapress.arizona.edu

ISBN-13: 978-0-8165-5316-7 (paperback)
ISBN-13: 978-0-8165-5317-4 (ebook)

Cover design by Leigh McDonald
Cover art by Lomayumtewa K. Ishii
Typeset by Sara Thaxton in 10/13.2 Adobe Caslon Pro with Museo Sans

Publication of this book is made possible in part by the proceeds of a permanent endowment created with the assistance of a Challenge Grant from the National Endowment for the Humanities, a federal agency.

Library of Congress Cataloging-in-Publication Data
Names: Jarratt-Snider, Karen, editor. | Nielsen, Marianne O., editor.
Title: Indigenous health and justice / edited by Karen Jarratt-Snider and Marianne O. Nielsen.
Other titles: Indigenous justice.
Description: Tucson : University of Arizona Press, 2024. | Series: Indigenous justice | Includes bibliographical references and index.
Identifiers: LCCN 2023024424 (print) | LCCN 2023024425 (ebook) | ISBN 9780816553167 (paperback) | ISBN 9780816553174 (ebook)
Subjects: LCSH: Indians of North America—Health and hygiene. | Indigenous peoples—Health and hygiene. | COVID-19 (Disease)—Social aspects. | Discrimination in medical care.
Classification: LCC RA448.5.I5 I543 2024 (print) | LCC RA448.5.I5 (ebook) | DDC 362.1089/97—dc23/eng/20231229
LC record available at https://lccn.loc.gov/2023024424
LC ebook record available at https://lccn.loc.gov/2023024425

Printed in the United States of America
♾ This paper meets the requirements of ANSI/NISO Z39.48-1992 (Permanence of Paper).

In memoriam Lomayumtewa Ishii,
Hopi father, husband, brother, scholar, and musician

This book is dedicated to the staff of the Indigenous
health and well-being centers operated by and for
Indigenous Peoples, nations, and communities. Your
services are invaluable, your dedication unquestioned.
May you continue for many generations to achieve
health justice for Indigenous Peoples.

A second dedication to this book is to all the
Indigenous people who have gone through health
trauma these last few years of pandemic, flu, RSV,
and emotional stress. Your resilience is an example
to us all.

CONTENTS

ACKNOWLEDGMENTS

MARIANNE AND KAREN would like to acknowledge the commitment of Northern Arizona University (NAU) to Indigenous students, nations, and communities that makes our work possible, and to NAU's College of Social and Behavioral Sciences for providing funding assistance to complete the previous book in the Indigenous Justice series. We would also like to acknowledge the patience of, and express our gratitude to, our authors and Kristen Buckles, editor-in-chief for the University of Arizona Press. Your faith in our ability to get this book done, come what may, has been humbling.

INDIGENOUS HEALTH
AND JUSTICE

INTRODUCTION

MARIANNE O. NIELSEN AND
KAREN JARRATT-SNIDER

O N JUNE 19, 2020, BrieAnna Frank of the *Arizona Republic* reported that the Navajo Police Department had lost its first officer to the COVID-19 pandemic. Officer Michael Lee was a longtime veteran of the department who started in 1990 as a recruit with the Navajo Police Academy. He was first stationed in Window Rock, Arizona, and finally in Chinle, Arizona, where he was felled by COVID-19 on the job, leaving behind a wife and children. Police chief Philip Francisco described the department as "devastated and heartbroken" and Navajo vice president Myron Lizer called Officer Lee "a truly honorable and distinguished person." Navajo President Jonathan Nez ordered the flags of the Navajo Nation to be lowered to half-mast in Lee's honor. His death would not be the last among first responders in Indian Country.

This book is about health injustices facing Indigenous individuals, communities, and nations, and the resilience they demonstrate in their efforts to create their own solutions to these injustices. Some chapters focus more on challenges created largely by the legacy of settler colonialism; others focus on the solutions and the strengths of Indigenous Peoples and communities in responding to these challenges. The COVID-19 pandemic is just one example both of the ongoing health disparity challenges and the fortitude of Indigenous Peoples and communities in meeting them.

As we were first editing this book, several variants of COVID-19 were causing yet another wave of infections throughout the United States and the world. At the beginning of the pandemic, Indigenous communities were hit particularly hard; the Navajo Nation, for example, had one of the highest infection and death rates in the country. Smaller Indigenous nations were equally if not harder hit. In New Mexico, for instance, Indigenous Peoples accounted for 8.8 percent of the state population but 60 percent of virus deaths (Manson and Buchwald 2021). Across the world, the pandemic focused public attention on the health inequities in Indigenous nations and communities.

The great majority of Indigenous communities acted effectively to protect their citizens, despite many challenges, such as lack of personal protective equipment (PPE) and testing, lack of running water for sanitization, multifamily homes that prevented physical distancing, limited access to medical services, understaffed health services, and delayed federal government funding (Manson and Buchwald 2021), along with a lack of Wi-Fi broadband for keeping people updated on the latest prevention strategies. Many tribal political and community leaders worked diligently to bring food, water, PPE, and vaccines to their communities. They counted on the communities of care that have been part of Indigenous cultures since time immemorial. While the COVID pandemic now mainly has become an endemic illness worldwide, its toll has been large and deep, and its consequences continue. Indigenous communities continue to prove their resilience every day, if not every hour, in dealing with its ongoing impacts.

COVID is just the latest in a long series of pandemics to affect Indigenous communities worldwide. Such pandemics have either been taken advantage of or inadequately responded to by colonial governments. Because of the extensive trade and communication networks of Indigenous Peoples, the early waves of disease started well before actual contact with settler colonists (Stannard 1992); yellow fever, bubonic plague, chicken pox, influenza, diphtheria, scarlet fever, typhoid fever, tuberculosis, measles, malaria, pertussis, dysentery, and, especially, smallpox, all had devastating results, sometimes killing up to 90 percent of the population (Manson and Buchwald 2021; Reading 2015; Stannard 1992; Shoemaker 1999). The first pandemics resulted from an absence of Indigenous immunity to European diseases, but a few settler-colonial leaders saw the potential of disease to deliberately remove Indigenous Peoples, and thus "infected blankets" were distributed in (likely unsuccessful) attempts at "germ warfare" (Ranlet 2000). Such epidemics contributed immensely to Indigenous social disorganization, cultural loss, family dissolution, and opportunistic government interventions—through, for example, removing children from their families to institutions as the government "awaited a cure" (Manson and Buchwald 2021). In addition, the colonization process over the next several hundred years (as has been well documented in many books and articles) led to malnutrition, starvation, coerced sterilization, torture, slavery, death, and debilitating poverty for many more Indigenous communities worldwide (Coates 2004, 129–35; Henry et al. 2018, 8–9).

An essential part of colonialism is to define the Indigenous inhabitants as inferior, primitive, savage, brutal, and inherently pathological (Trigger 1985; Reading 2015). According to first the Catholic Church and then others invested in missionary work, Indigenous Peoples were pagans whose souls needed to be saved, even at the cost of ruining their health, when missionaries were not actually killing the potential converts. Later colonial ideologies began to rely on social Darwinism. It was not the fault of the settler colonists, to the settler colonists' way of thinking, if Indigenous Peoples were not fit to survive when faced with the "bolder, brighter, better" Europeans (Blaut 1993). They were considered to be a dying race undeserving, indeed, un-needing of equitable opportunities (Fixico 2013). Victim blaming of Indigenous populations has been a constant throughout colonization, with settler colonists focused on stereotypes of "dirty" and "illiterate" Indigenous populations rather than acknowledging the horrendous conditions under which most Indigenous Peoples lived during disease epidemics and on reservations (Manson and Buchwald 2021). Reading (2015, 7) writes that in Canada, "Western medicine played a key role in the colonization of Indigenous peoples. . . . For the most part, early Indigenous health policy was based on notions of 'white' racial superiority, assimilation goals, and an irrational fear of 'interracial' contagion."

Such disregard for the health of the original inhabitants of Indigenous lands has had negative consequences on their physical, mental, spiritual, and emotional health, and this attitude has been carried on in colonial legislation and institutions that continue to oppress and structurally discriminate against Indigenous Peoples today (Kirmayer et al. 2011). This enduring racism is evident in the lack of adequate funding (Reading 2015) and the limits placed on Indigenous self-determination to operate culturally sensitive health programs. For example, writing about the Inuit, Kirmayer et al. (2011, 88) state that "resilience is not so much about adaptation to the Arctic environment but ongoing efforts to adapt to a daunting social environment created by the incongruent and conflicting policies and institutions introduced by southern administration."

Actions by various governments in colonized countries have contributed to serious health problems that continue today. As the special rapporteur on the rights of Indigenous Peoples (UNOHCHR 2020) stated, "I am receiving more reports every day from all corners of the globe about how Indigenous communities are affected by the COVID-19 pandemic, and it deeply worries me to see it is not always about health issues." He mentions reports of Indigenous Peoples being denied freedom of association and expression, corporations invading Indigenous lands to take their resources, environmental impact statements for Indigenous lands being cancelled, and huge extractive and infrastructure projects receiving government permission to operate on Indigenous lands—all justified by corporate and governmental entities as being necessary due to COVID-19. The consequences have been and continue to be immense. As the UNOHCHR points out, "Indigenous peoples who lose their lands and livelihoods are pushed further into poverty, higher rates of malnutrition, lack of access to clean water and sanitation, as well as exclusion from medical services, which in turn renders them particularly vulnerable to disease."

Forced relocation not only removes Indigenous Peoples from their spiritual homes but from their traditional food and water sources (Henry et al. 2018, 9; Reading 2015). In the United States, state-facilitated uranium mining and other forms of environmental degradation contaminating the earth, water, and air led to the Diné people, for instance, having some of the highest cancer rates in the country (Jarratt-Snider and Nielsen 2020). Such environmental contaminants are also an issue for Indigenous Peoples in other colonized countries; many Aboriginal communities in Canada, for example, must survive heavy metals and PCBs (polychlorinated biphenyls) in their water and food (Waldram, Herring, and Young 2006, 116). These conditions have been worsened by climate change that has led to the disappearance of Indigenous lands and the foodstuffs and medicines they contained. As a report by the Status of Tribes and Climate Change Working Group states, "Given close relationships with the natural world stemming from deep spiritual and cultural connections and subsistence lifeways, Indigenous peoples are on the frontlines of those experiencing and adapting to climate change" (STACC Working Group 2021, 6). Hunt, Estus, and Walker (2021) also discuss the reduction in traditional food sources due to lost land. They quote a Houma Indian citizen on this matter: "I don't like the idea of having to leave but I don't want to go through another storm. Climate change is definitely causing this. People who deny that need a lesson in science." The Indigenous Peoples of Alaska face similar problems: "Dead fish have been found on the Tanana River and changes in caribou migration present new challenges for subsistence hunters," and flooding, fires, and drought caused by climate change have affected the health of Indigenous people across the United States (Hunt, Estus, and Walker 2021). On the more positive side, Companion (2023), in another volume in this series, describes how food sovereignty movements in three Indigenous groups in the United States are working to help Indigenous communities survive climate change.

It is not just large-scale crises caused by state-corporate actions that have contributed to the poor health of Indigenous Peoples. Day-to-day institutional racism also contributes through, for instance, the U.S. government's issuance of high-saturated-fat, low-fiber, high-carbohydrate, and highly processed "commodity foods" that are linked to obesity and diabetes. Known by its formal title, the Food Distribution Program on Indian Reservations, this U.S. Department of Agriculture program now offers more healthy choices in some areas (USDA 2020), but for decades, commodity foods consisted of white rice, granulated sugar, powdered milk, powdered eggs, lard, beans, processed cheese-like products, and a highly processed product labeled simply as "canned meat" (as Jarratt-Snider personally observed from 1965 to 1978). The only fruits or vegetables included were the dried beans and an occasional can of grape juice. The lack of access to healthy food because of reservation "food deserts" (no nearby supermarkets or grocery stores), and the lack of access to well-funded and culturally appropriate health-care facilities (see the chapter by Dietrich and Schroedel), are also major contributors. Indigenous Peoples still encounter intentional or unintentional racism and a lack of knowledge about Indigenous culture (Manson and Buchwald 2021; USCCR 2004). Indigenous individuals may be discriminated against and blamed if they seek health services as the victim of, for example, a serious disease, family violence, or sexual assault (Manson and Buchwald 2021; Amnesty International 2007).

Yet, despite these persistent challenges, Indigenous Peoples and communities are still here and have been fighting to maintain and regain their resilience and health. Food sovereignty movements have sprung up in Indigenous communities across the country, as have culturally sensitive health and disease prevention and education programs, horticultural initiatives, and mental well-being programs. Indigenous-run health clinics are relatively common. Our home base of Flagstaff, Arizona, for instance, has two: the Native Americans for Community Action Family Health Center, which provides mental health, community development, and illness prevention programs in addition to medical services (NACA, n.d.); and the Sacred Peaks Health Center (which provides psychological services, physical therapy, and health education in addition to medical services) (Tuba City 2023). Note the holistic nature of these services.

Indigenous health organizations are rooted in the values and history of Indigenous cultures, and therefore, they are more likely to provide culturally appropriate and effective services (Nielsen and Brown 2012). Another such example is how the Cherokee Nation has asserted its self-determination by taking more and more control of its health-care facilities and systems (as the chapter by Begay, Petillo, and Goldtooth discusses). Not only does the nation offer a breadth of health-care services, but they also have several outpatient clinics, and in 2018, they assumed control of the W. W. Hastings Hospital (Cherokee Nation 2021). A third example is recent research in Canada that explored the impact of Indigenous urban youths' relationship with land on their perspectives of their own mental and physical health and resilience (Hatala et al. 2020).

WHAT ARE INDIGENOUS SOCIAL DETERMINANTS OF HEALTH?

Indigenous determinants of health (IDOH) are not the same as the commonly known social determinants of health, although they overlap. The U.S. Department of Health and Human Services (n.d.) places the social determinants of health in five "domains": economic stability, education access and quality, health-care access and quality, neighborhood and built environment, and social and community context. Their goal for economic stability, for example, is to "help people earn steady incomes that allow them to meet their health needs." Their goal for health-care access and quality is to "increase access to comprehensive, high-quality health care services" which has objectives addressing adolescents, cancer, children, community, drug and alcohol use, family planning, health care, health communication, health information technology, health insurance, oral conditions, people with disabilities, pregnancy and childbirth, sensory or communication disorders, sexually transmitted diseases, and other topics. All of these are issues shared between Indigenous and non-Indigenous communities, both nationally and internationally.

While Indigenous Peoples worldwide have the greatest disparities in health, and identify the impacts of colonialism as the primary fundamental determinant (de Leeuw, Lindsay, and Greenwood 2015), Indigenous nations' and their communities' responses to these disparities are examples of strength and resilience. IDOH recognize the tragic impacts that colonization has had on the well-being of Indigenous individual and communities. As Wilson and Richmond (2009, 367) write, "Current patterns of health and social suffering reflect the combined effects of colonial oppression, systemic racism, and discrimination as well as unequal access to human, social, and environmental resources. Such inequalities in health and well-being have been attributed to the ongoing legacies of colonialism." These patterns are evident in the majority of Indigenous populations worldwide (Wilson and Richmond 2009).

Reading (2015) points out that there are three levels of IDOH— proximal, intermediate, and distal. Her analysis of diabetes in Canadian Indigenous populations illustrates the importance of these distinctions:

If we hope to appropriately address diabetes, we must first understand what determinants are influencing the development and persistence of this debilitating and life-threatening illness. Yet, if we limit our analysis to its proximal determinants, as is often the case, we will continue to focus our attention on obesity, poor diet, and sedentary lifestyle. If, however, we explore further, we will likely encounter additional determinants such as economic (lack of resources to afford healthy food) and/or geographic (remote locations with expensive shipping costs) barriers to accessing healthy market or country foods, as well as physical environments that do not always support health-promoting exercise (crowded housing, lack of sidewalks or walking trails, cold weather, lack of accessible recreational infrastructure or programs). . . . If we search deeper still for the determinants responsible for shaping these conditions, we discover the root of the problem—a colonial structure—fashioned from the centralization of Aboriginal peoples into remote communities and reserves, the oppressive nature of the Indian Act, the damaging legacy of residential schools, racial discrimination in social environments and the labour market, as well as lack of public or private investment in economic development for Aboriginal communities.

IDOH go beyond what non-Indigenous scholars see as "social" to include relations with the land and the environment, spirituality, history, language and culture, and systems of knowledge (de Leeuw, Lindsay, and Greenwood 2015). For example, a recent "first of its kind" wellness tool "measures how cultural interventions affect a person's wellness from a whole person and strengths-based view" (Thunderbird Partnership Foundation 202). As de Leeuw, Lindsay, and Greenwood (2015, xiii) write, "There are a great variety of determinants of Indigenous Peoples' health. These include, to name a few, geographic determinants, economic determinants, historical determinants, narrative and genealogical determinants, and structural determinants—most of which are not individually or biologically dictated, but all of which are unique because they interface with and are impacted by colonialism of the past and the present." Kirmayer et al. (2011, 85) writing about Canada, agree, adding to factors already mentioned "the subsequent efforts of extermination, marginalization, or exclusion, and, eventually, state dependency . . . other regimes of cultural suppression and forced assimilation; experiences of racism and discrimination and the negative portrayal of Aboriginal people in the dominant society; and the importance of relationship to the land or place for individual and communal identity." Both the historical effects and the continuing effects of colonization contribute to Indigenous Peoples' health disparities. Brave Heart (1998, 1999) articulated the effects of the generations of colonial violence ranging from the boarding schools to the current issues related to murdered and missing Indigenous persons. These resulted in historical trauma, a contributing factor to Indigenous health disparities in mental wellness. Historical trauma, such as violence associated with the early stage of colonialism, is an example of distal trauma, whereas the COVID pandemic offers an example of proximate trauma.

Recently, Gone et al. (2019) examined over thirty studies involving Indigenous historical trauma and health, and while there were three different types of studies included in the review, the authors concluded that "many studies reported statistically significant associations between higher indicators of [Indigenous historical trauma] and adverse health outcomes." Most Indigenous conceptions of physical, mental, spiritual, environmental, and other aspects of health are centered on the concepts of harmony, interconnectedness, and balance, whether these are represented in the medicine wheel of many North American Indigenous Peoples, the whole community view of Native Hawaiians, or the four house walls metaphor of Māori people (Wilson and Richmond 2009). This balance in many North American Indigenous cultures refers to harmony within the individual but also to a much broader harmony—between individuals and the environment, their community, and the spirit world. For example, among the Canadian Inuit, "these concepts are captured within *inuuqatigiittiarniq*, which depends on the balance and harmony of economic, cultural, environmental, and biological factors. A careful balance of factors manifests as *inummarik*—a most genuine person—in a continuous lifelong process of developing interaction with people and animals, community and environment" (Wilson and Richmond 2009, 366). The Diné people have the concept of *hózhó*, which Austin describes as a condition encompassing "everything that Navajos consider positive and good; positive characteristics that Navajos believe contribute to living life to the fullest. These positive characteristics include beauty, harmony, goodness, happiness, right social relations, *good health*, and acquisition of knowledge" (emphasis added). *Hózhó* includes everything "tangible and intangible . . . in its proper place and functioning well with everything else." This "everything" refers to the "interconnected, interrelated, and interdependent elements . . . that form a unified whole" (Austin 2009, 54).

As noted above, in keeping with the holistic and interconnected world view of Indigenous Peoples, health is not simply defined as physical health, as it has been until recently in most non-Indigenous societies. Indigenous cultures believe in balance so that health is more than physical and mental; it is also emotional and spiritual (Bopp et al. 1988). Additionally, the health needs of Indigenous subpopulations are acknowledged. This includes the reproductive health of women, the health of youth and children, and the health of families and whole communities.

INDIGENOUS HEALTH WORLDWIDE

According to the director-general of the World Health Organization, Dr. Tedros Adhanom Ghebreyesus (2017), "health is a fundamental human right." He goes on to say that "the enjoyment of the highest attainable standard of health is one of the fundamental rights of every human being without distinction of race, religion, political belief, economic or social condition." He further states:

- The right to health for all people means that everyone should have access to the health services they need, when and where they need them, without suffering financial hardship.
- No one should get sick and die because they are poor, or because they cannot access the health services they need.
- The right to health also means that everyone should be entitled to control their own health and body, including having access to sexual and reproductive information and services, free from violence and discrimination.
- Good health is also clearly determined by other basic human rights including access to safe drinking water and sanitation, nutritious food, adequate housing, education and safe working conditions.

Also according to Ghebreyesus (2017), "When people are marginalized or face stigma or discrimination, their physical and mental health suffers. Discrimination in health care is unacceptable and is a major barrier to development." Nevertheless, the government of many colonized countries have failed to live up to WHO aspirations. This is very likely the result of continuing colonial ideologies that see Indigenous Peoples as inferior and primitive, and that support the acquisitive path to the "proper" usage of natural resources by corporations, aided and abetted by colonial governments. Settler-colonist greed originally drove colonialism, and settler colonists saw the need to "replace" Indigenous populations either by extermination or assimilation (Wolfe 2006).

State-corporate crimes have been committed in order to take Indigenous Peoples' resources away from them, such as fraud in treaty making (and breaking), violence to remove Indigenous Peoples from their land, and the desecration of sacred sites (see Nielsen and Robyn 2019). Great social harms have been committed against Indigenous Peoples that have led to historical trauma and internalized violence (e.g., suicide, substance abuse) and externalized violence (e.g., family violence, sexual assault, homicide), according to Native American psychologists Eduardo and Bonnie Duran (1995). Historical trauma can be linked to significant health issues for children, such as child maltreatment (Federal Interagency Forum 2022), and for women, such as lack of access to prenatal care (Ali-Joseph and McCue 2023). Indigenous Peoples have health issues now that were rare or didn't exist before colonialism, such as family/domestic violence, substance abuse, and suicide.

Because of colonial legal impositions and depopulation though disease and violence, traditional health interventions were given little time to adapt, but these adaptations are now being implemented. Manson and Buchwald, writing about the COVID pandemic, describe the use of traditional medicines to address certain COVID symptoms, to boost immunological systems, and to encourage self-care. In addition, "biomedical practitioners have joined with traditional healers to demonstrate how current forms of mitigation, such as handwashing, social distancing, and wearing masks, can enable the latter to safely practice their healing rituals" (Manson and Buchwald 2021). They also give examples of Indigenous youth caring for elders, and Indigenous-operated restaurants preparing meals of traditional food for urban-based elderly Native individuals. The incorporation of traditional Indigenous knowledge is essential for the success of these strategies.

Some Indigenous communities have developed "hybrid" healing programs, in partnership with Western-based medical interventions, that have proven successful, such as substance abuse, intervention, and recovery programs. For example, Poundmaker's Lodge Treatment Centres, a Canadian substance abuse treatment facility, has provided services since 1973. Their website states, "Through concepts based in the cultural and spiritual beliefs of traditional First Nations, Metis and Inuit peoples in combination with 12-Step, abstinence based recovery, Poundmaker's Lodge also offers opioid treatment and an Indigenous wholistic treatment experience that focuses on the root causes of addiction and empowers people in their recovery from addiction" (n.d.).

Such Indigenous service organizations can be found in many colonized countries. For example, the Pangula Mannamurna Aboriginal Corporation (n.d.) in Mount Gamber, South Australia, provides not only medical services but programs focusing on social-emotional well-being and parenting, as well as a women's crafts program and a children's play group. Tuu Oho Mai Services, formerly called the Hamilton Abuse Intervention Program in Aotearoa / New Zealand, described in the chapter by Dodd and Nielsen, provides education about family violence prevention, operates a crisis hotline, and offers advocacy in court.

Recent legal decisions have made the practice of de facto sovereignty less of a struggle in some areas of the world. For example, in the United States, in 2021, the U.S. Court of Appeals for the Eighth Circuit ruled that as found in the Treaty of Fort Laramie (1868), health services were a treaty right of the Rosebud Sioux (Pember 2021). Federally funded health care to American Indians has been part of many treaties and laws, such as the Snyder Act (1921) and Indian Health Care Improvement Act (2010). Originally, treaty language was included to push American Indian nations toward Western medicine and away from traditional health care. According to Pember, "In ruling that competent health care is a treaty right, however, the [Eighth Circuit] court imbues it with the power of the U.S. Constitution in which treaty rights are considered to be the supreme law of the land." Note the emphasis on *competent* health care. The ruling points out that the federal Indian Health Service (IHS) needs to provide more than the minimum services. Pember notes that the IHS spends $3,779 per user compared to Medicaid, which spends $8,093 per user. The IHS (2020) reports slightly higher numbers, with $4,078 per American Indian user, compared to the U.S. national health expenditure of $9,726 per user. Such disparities in funding have led to serious disparities in health-care access. The 2021 ruling was the result of the *Rosebud Sioux Tribe v. United States* case that was filed in 2016 after the IHS closed the only emergency room on the reservation, forcing tribal members to travel over fifty miles for help; the ruling read, in part, "The Treaty created a duty . . . for the government to provide competent, physician-led health care to the tribe and its members. We affirm" (Pember 2021).

In the United States, state-recognized nations have similar problems with acquiring access to the funding they need to operate their own services, due to their lack of access to federal funding and the reluctance of many states to invest in Indian Country health. While rulings such as the one in the Rosebud Sioux case have the potential to give tribal nations more leverage in pursuing increased funding from Congress for health-care services (Pember 2021), some state governments have actively fought nation-based COVID prevention, for example, as occurred in South Dakota (Manson and Buchwald 2021).

Worldwide, Indigenous Peoples are understandably "suspicious of promises of aid that have often proved to be hollow offerings" (Manson and Buchwald 2021) In other words, many Indigenous nations and communities, occasionally with legal support, have actively sought greater control over their lives and their communities. In the case of overcoming health issues, they have developed their own services—that is, they are practicing de facto sovereignty. They are taking control "on the ground" of solutions to the issues created by colonialism both in the past and today.

DE FACTO SOVEREIGNTY, HEALTH, AND RESILIENCE

Poor access to health care and other resources have led many Indigenous nations and urban populations to develop their own health-care services, some of which are healing centers that provide Western-style medical personnel (doctors, nurses, nutritionists, for example) alongside traditional healers (Wilson and Richmond 2009). These efforts contribute to de facto self-determination, which we have defined as "the practice of Indigenous Peoples and communities asserting authority by developing programs and services that address some of the many social justice issues" that affect them (Jarratt-Snider and Nielsen 2018, 191). The practice of de facto sovereignty is just one of many through which Indigenous Peoples have been demonstrating their resilience. Settler colonists and colonial governments have been underestimating the resilience of Indigenous Peoples and individuals for centuries (Fixico 2013). Kirmayer et al. (2011, 84) define resilience as "the ability to do well despite adversity" and explain that it is "a dynamic process of social and psychological adaptation and transformation. As such, resilience can be a characteristic of individuals, families, communities, or larger social groups and is manifested as positive outcomes in the face of historical and current stresses" (85).

Resilience is key to Indigenous health because its foundation is cultural values and knowledge that have "persisted despite historical adversity or have emerged out of the renewal of indigenous identities . . . [that] include culturally distinctive concepts of the person, the importance of collective history, the richness of Aboriginal languages and traditions, and the importance of individual and collective agency and activism" (Kirmayer et al. 2011, 88).

Resilience research has tended to focus on individual adaptability, but this is insufficient because of the collectivist nature of most Indigenous cultures. New resilience research takes into account individual interconnections with family, community, environment, and spiritual beings. As Kirmayer et al. write, "Indigenous concepts provide ways to approach a dynamic, systemic, ecological view of resilience." They also point out that certain Indigenous determinants of health are related to sources of resilience: "Some of these strategies of resilience draw from traditional knowledge, values and practices, but they also reflect ongoing responses to the new challenges posed by evolving relationships with the dominant society and emerging global networks of indigenous peoples pursuing common cause" (2011, 85). They assert that the types of resilience shown by individuals vary depending on factors such as their life history, age, gender, and degree of education that may change over time, and are rooted in the history and environments of the specific Indigenous Peoples (86).

Other resources available to Indigenous Peoples include strengthening their links with other Indigenous communities in the same region (Kirmayer et al. 2011) and globally (Nielsen and Robyn 2019).

CONCLUSION

Colonial oppression, systemic racism, discrimination, and poor access to a wide range of resources detract from Indigenous health and contribute to continuing health inequities (Wilson and Richmond 2009). These factors have contributed to structural inadequacies that in turn have created circular challenges such as chronic underfunding, understaffing, and culturally insensitive health-care provision. Nevertheless, Indigenous Peoples are working actively to end such legacies and to prove their resilience. Donald Fixico (2013, 15) writes that "resilience is required of anyone who wishes to survive. . . . Resilience offers hope to a dismal future . . . . Resilience is the ability to recover from a dire situation, and it is an essential step toward rebuilding." Indigenous Peoples are rebuilding the health of their members, communities, and nations.

THEMES

The chapters in this volume address this **resilience** (one of the key themes of this book) as well as Indigenous health disparities and communities' and nations' solutions and responses to these issues (see the chapters by Camplain et al.; Paquin; Haskie; Thompson and Marek-Martinez; Dodd and Nielsen). In many cases, these solutions to health injustice are examples of de facto sovereignty and self-determination. **Health justice is a holistic concept** that encompasses all aspects of the world in which Indigenous Peoples survive and thrive. As Thompson and Marek-Martinez point out, Indigenous health is a concept that encompasses healthy relationships (a "complex living system") among land, the water, the environment, the spirits, the communities, and the beings who live in all of them. On another note, Paquin (chapter 3) relates the importance of education to health and justice.

It is therefore not surprising that a prominent theme shared by all chapters is understanding **the ongoing impacts of colonialism** on the health of Indigenous individuals and communities. These impacts take a wide variety of forms, including economic, political, and social marginalization, and lead to many types of violence, disease, and mortality (as discussed by most authors in this volume). To this list can be added jurisdictional issues (Camplain et al.) and the federal government's inadequate support of health-care services through its refusal, delay, or inability to live up to its **trust responsibility** to Indigenous Peoples, and what that has meant in terms of disproportionate disease and death rates (Camplain et al.; Dietrich and Schroedel; Kunze and Camarillo). These chapters point to an overarching theme of the **structural and institutional racism** that exists in federal American Indian policy in the area of health care. This racism is particularly apparent in the book's section on COVID-19, though the emphasis of the book is on the resilient, innovative, and timely responses of Indigenous communities and nations (Begay, Petillo, and Goldtooth; Haskie; and Kunze and Camarillo). **Resilience in the face of COVID** is another theme of this book.

Just as it has been in past volumes, an overall theme in this volume is **de facto sovereignty** and its role in decolonizing health services. The adaptability and flexibility of Indigenous Peoples in resolving issues when colonial governments are too slow, too uncaring, or too hobbled by politics to act are demonstrated in all of the chapters. For example, Dietrich and Schroedel discuss this in terms of nations developing alternatives to inadequate IHS care; Begay, Petillo, and Goldtooth discuss responses to the COVID pandemic by American Indigenous governments; Camplain et al. and Haskie, respectively, describe the collaboration between Indigenous and non-Indigenous government health services for incarcerated Indigenous people in the American Southwest, and in responding to the pandemic; Thompson and Marek-Martinez write about reclaiming relationships with the land and the community through the use of Indigenous protocols; and Dodd and Nielsen describe the cultural development and operation of an Indigenous-run health organization that specializes in preventing domestic violence in Aotearoa / New Zealand.

Health care is identified as a basic **human and American constitutional right** by Camplain et al., as is the need for health care for both physical and mental issues. Numerous authors in this book explore the **use of law** as a tool to improve health services (Camplain et al.; Dietrich and Schroedel; Kunze and Camarillo; Begay, Petillo, and Goldtooth) as well as the conflict that occurs between American federal and state law, on the one hand, and tribal laws and regulations on the other (Kunze and Camarillo). **Politics and political leaders play an impactful role**, either interfering in the provision of health-care services, as Kunze and Camarillo mention in the case of state law, or using creative problem-solving to improve not only health-care delivery (Haskie) but tribal sovereignty, as explored by Begay, Petillo, and Goldtooth.

As was discussed at length in the most recent volume in this series, *Indigenous Gender and Justice* (Nielsen and Jarratt-Snider 2023), Camplain et al. also point out how health-care disparities **particularly affect Indigenous women** and how their health-caring roles can make them more susceptible to disease (Haskie). Yet Indigenous women also play a vital role in connecting Indigenous Peoples to the land and the health-related resources the land provides (Thompson and Marek-Martinez). Begay, Petillo, and Goldtooth also point out how inadequate health-care responses, as occurred with the COVID pandemic, can have serious repercussions that include the loss of traditional knowledge holders and, hence, ceremonies and language. Yet the **use of cultural resources** spread through oral tradition, health programs, and other means is needed to make health-care services as effective as possible (Begay, Petillo, and Goldtooth; Thompson and Marek-Martinez; Dodd and Nielsen). The importance of connections to the environment and spirituality are particularly noted by Thompson and Marek-Martinez, and Dodd and Nielsen.

Kunze and Camarillo emphasize the issue of **inaccurate and inadequate media portrayals** of Indigenous Peoples and communities. They specifically point out the impact that these inaccuracies and stereotyping portrayals can have on the public and government decision-makers tasked with providing funding and other resources for health care. Haskie on the other hand points out the important role that **media can play in disseminating information** about the prevention of disease and resources available to fight it, and the need for more public health information. **Indigenous responses to globalization** are also noted (Begay, Petillo, and Goldtooth; Dodd and Nielsen), for example the fact that Indigenous Peoples can more easily share information and strategies in the twenty-first century, such as effective responses to COVID.

A final theme that several authors explore is the **need for more research** in the many areas of health care for Indigenous Peoples (Camplain et al.; Kunze and Camarillo).

THE BOOK

Indigenous Health and Justice is the fifth volume in the Indigenous Justice series from the University of Arizona Press. The series is edited by Karen Jarratt-Snider and Marianne O. Nielsen. We have a combined sixty-eight years of experience in engaged research with Indigenous communities and nations worldwide. Individually and together, we have published a great many peer-reviewed articles, book chapters, and research reports, as well as books outside of this series. We have served as consultants to Indigenous nations; agencies at the county, state, provincial, and federal levels; and service organizations in the United States, Canada, and Australia.

Each volume in the series focuses on different aspects of the many kinds of justice that affect Indigenous Peoples, mainly in the United States but also in other colonized countries. As mentioned earlier, this volume contains information on Canada and Aotearoa. Indigenous Peoples in Africa, Latin America, Asia, and elsewhere are not represented in this particular volume; the issues in these areas, and Indigenous responses to them, could easily fill several volumes.

REFERENCES

Ali-Joseph, Alisse, and Kelly McCue. 2023. "Breastfeeding and Indigenous Reproductive Justice." In *Indigenous Justice and Gender*, edited by Marianne O. Nielsen and Karen Jarratt-Snider, 25–41. Tucson: University of Arizona Press.

Amnesty International. 2007. *Maze of Injustice: The Failure to Protect Indigenous Women from Sexual Violence in the USA*. https://www.amnesty.org/en/wp-content /uploads/2021/05/AMR510352007ENGLISH.pdf.

Austin, Raymond D. 2009. *Navajo Courts and Common Law: A Tradition of Tribal Self-Governance*. Minneapolis: University of Minnesota Press.

Blaut, J. M. 1993. *The Colonizer's Model of the World*. New York: Guilford Press.

Bopp, Julie, Michael Bopp, Phil Lane, and Carolyn Peter. 1988. *The Sacred Tree*. Rev. ed. Lethbridge, AB: Four Worlds Development.

Brave Heart, Maria Yellow Horse. 1998. "The Return to The Sacred Path: Healing the Historical Trauma and Historical Unresolved Grief Response Among the Lakota Through a Psychoeducational Group Intervention." *Smith College Studies in Social Work* 68, no. 3: 287–305. https://doi.org/10.1080/00377319809517532.

Brave Heart, Maria Yellow Horse. 1999. "Gender Differences in the Historical Trauma Response Among the Lakota." *Journal of Health and Social Policy* 10, no. 4: 1–21. https://doi.org/10.1300/J045v10n04_01.

Cherokee Nation. 2021. "Health Services." Last updated August 26, 2021. https:// health.cherokee.org/health-center-and-hospital-locations/.

Coates, Ken S. 2004. *A Global History of Indigenous Peoples: Struggle and Survival*. New York: Palgrave Macmillan.

Companion, Michéle. 2023. "Culture Work in a Changing Climate: Using Food Sovereignty Movements to Rebuild the Future." In *Indigenous Justice and Gender*, edited by Marianne O. Nielsen and Karen Jarratt-Snider, 149–77. Tucson: University of Arizona Press.

de Leeuw, Sarah, Nicole M. Lindsay, and Margo Greenwood. 2015. "Rethinking Determinants of Indigenous Peoples' Health in Canada." In *Determinants of Indigenous Peoples' Health in Canada: Beyond the Social*, edited by Margo Greenwood, Sarah de Leeuw, Nicole Marie Lindsay, and Charlotte Reading, xi–xxix. Toronto: Canadian Scholars.

Duran, Eduardo, and Bonnie Duran. 1995. *Native American Postcolonial Psychology*. New York: SUNY Press.

Federal Interagency Forum on Child and Family Statistics. 2022. *America's Children in Brief: Key National Indicators of Well-Being, 2022*. Washington, D.C.: U.S. Government Printing Office. https://www.childstats.gov/pdf/ac2022/ac_22.pdf.

Fixico, Donald. 2013. *Indian Resilience and Rebuilding: Indigenous Nations in the Modern American West*. Tucson: University of Arizona Press.

Frank, BrieAnna J. 2020. "Navajo Police Department Officer Dies of COVID-19, Marking Department's 1st Line-of-Duty Death from Pandemic." *Arizona Republic*, June 19, 2020. https://www.azcentral.com/story/news/local/arizona/2020/06/19/navajo-police-department-officer-dies-covid-19-first-line-duty-death/3223305001/.

Ghebreyesus, Tedros Adhanom. 2017. "Health Is a Fundamental Human Right." World Health Organization. Commentary. December 10, 2017. https://www.who.int/news-room/commentaries/detail/health-is-a-fundamental-human-right.

Gone, Joseph P., W. E. Hartmann, A. Pomerville, D. C. Wendt, S. H. Klern, and R. L. Burrage. 2019. "The Impact of Historical Trauma on Health Outcomes for Indigenous Populations in the USA and Canada: A Systematic Review." *American Psychologist* 74, no. 1: 20–35. https://doi.org/10.1037/amp0000338

Hatala, Andrew R., Chinyere Njeze, Darrien Morton, Tamara Pearl, and Kelley Bird-Naytowhow. 2020. "Land and Nature as Sources of Health and Resilience Among Indigenous Youth in an Urban Canadian Context: A Photovoice Exploration." *BMC Public Health* 20: 538–52. https://doi.org/10.1186/s12889-020-08647-z.

Henry, Robert, Amanda LaVallee, Nancy Van Styvendall, and Roberta A. Innes. 2018. "Introduction." In *Global Indigenous Health*, edited by Robert Henry, Amanda LaVallee, Nancy Van Styvendall, and Robert A. Innes, 3–24. Tucson: University of Arizona Press.

Hunt, Dianna, Joaqlin Estus, and Richard A. Walker. 2021. "Homelands in Peril." *Indian Country Today*, October 27, 2021. https://indiancountrytoday.com/news/homelands-in-peril.

IHS (U.S. Indian Health Service). 2020. "IHS Profile." https://www.ihs.gov/newsroom/factsheets/ihsprofile/.

Jarratt-Snider, Karen, and Marianne O. Nielsen. 2018. "Conclusion." In *Crime and Social Justice in Indian Country*, edited by Marianne O. Nielsen and Karen Jarratt-Snider, 185–93. Tucson: University of Arizona Press.

Jarratt-Snider, Karen, and Marianne O. Nielsen, eds. 2020. *Indigenous Environmental Justice*. Tucson: University of Arizona Press.

Kirmayer, Laurence J., Stéphane Dandeneau, Elizabeth Marshall, Morgan Kahentonni Phillips, and Karla Jessen Williamson. 2011. "Rethinking Resilience from Indigenous Perspectives." *Canadian Journal of Psychiatry* 56, no. 2: 84–91. https://doi.org/10.1177/07067437110560020.

Manson, Spero M., and Dedra Buchwald. 2021. "Bringing Light to the Darkness: COVID-19 and Survivance of American Indians and Alaska Natives." *Health Equity* 5, no. 1 (February): 59–63. https://doi.org/10.1089/heq.2020.0123.

NACA (Native Americans for Community Action). n.d. "Family Health." https://nacainc.org/family-health/.

Nielsen, Marianne O., and Samantha Brown. 2012. "Beyond Justice: What Makes an Indigenous Justice Organization?" *American Indian Culture and Research Journal* 36, no. 2: 47–73. https://doi.org/10.17953/aicr.36.2.m7441vm524166442.

Nielsen, Marianne O., and Karen Jarratt-Snider, eds. 2023. *Indigenous Justice and Gender.* Tucson: University of Arizona Press.

Nielsen, Marianne O., and Linda M. Robyn. 2019. *Colonialism Is Crime.* New Brunswick, NJ: Rutgers University Press.

Pangula Mannamurna Aboriginal Corporation. n.d. "Services." Accessed May 26, 2023. http://pangula.org.au/services/.

Pember, Mary Annette. 2021. "Federal Court Affirms Health Care as Treaty Right." *Indian Country Today*, September 1, 2021. https://indiancountrytoday.com/news/federal-court-affirms-health-care-as-treaty-right.

Poundmaker's Lodge Treatment Centres. n.d. "Home." Accessed May 26, 2023. https://poundmakerslodge.ca/.

Ranlet, Philip. 2000. "The British, the Indians, and Smallpox: What Actually Happened at Fort Pitt in 1763?" *Pennsylvania History: A Journal of Mid-Atlantic Studies* 67, no. 3 (Summer): 427–41. https://www.jstor.org/stable/27774278.

Reading, Charlotte. 2015. "Structural Determinants of Aboriginal Peoples' Health." In *Determinants of Indigenous Peoples' Health in Canada: Beyond the Social,* edited by Margo Greenwood, Sarah de Leeuw, Nicole M. Lindsay, and Charlotte Reading, 3–15. Toronto: Canadian Scholars.

Shoemaker, Nancy. 1999. *American Indian Population Recovery in the Twentieth Century.* Albuquerque: University of New Mexico Press.

STACC (Status of Tribes and Climate Change) Working Group. 2021. *Status of Tribes and Climate Change Report.* Flagstaff: Institute for Tribal Environmental Professionals, Northern Arizona University. http://nau.edu/stacc2021.

Stannard, David E. 1992. *American Holocaust: The Conquest of the New World.* New York: Oxford University Press.

Thunderbird Partnership Foundation. n.d. "Native Wellness Assessment (NWA)." Accessed May 29, 2023. https://thunderbirdpf.org/native-wellness-assessment/.

Trigger, Bruce G. 1985. *Natives and Newcomers: Canada's "Heroic Age" Reconsidered.* Montreal: McGill University Press.

Tuba City (Tuba City Regional health Care Corporation). 2023. "Services at Sacred Peaks." https://tchealth.org/sacredpeaks/services.html.

UNOHCHR (United Nations Office of the High Commissioner for Human Rights). 2020. "'COVID-19 Is Devastating Indigenous Communities Worldwide, and It's Not Only About Health'—UN Expert Warns." Press release. May 18, 2020. https://www.ohchr.org/EN/NewsEvents/Pages/DisplayNews .aspx?NewsID=25893&LangID=E.

USCCR (U.S. Commission on Civil Rights). 2004. *Broken Promises: Evaluating the Native American Health Care System.* https://www.usccr.gov/files/pubs/docs /nabroken.pdf.

USDA (U.S. Department of Agriculture). 2020. "Food Distribution Program on Indian Reservations." Fact sheet. January 2020. https://fns-prod.azureedge .us/sites/default/files/resource-files/fdpir-program-fact-sheet-2020-for%20 website.pdf.

U.S. Department of Health and Human Services. n.d. "Healthy People 2030: Social Determinants of Health." Office of Disease Prevention and Health Promotion. Accessed October 13, 2021. https://health.gov/healthypeople/objec tives-and-data/social-determinants-health.

Waldram, James B., D. Ann Herring, and T. Kue Young. 2006. *Aboriginal Health in Canada: Historical, Cultural, and Epidemiological Perspectives.* 2nd ed. Toronto: University of Toronto Press.

Wilson, K., and C. Richmond. 2009. "Indigenous Health and Medicine." In *International Encyclopedia of Human Geography*, edited by Rob Kitchen and Nigel Thrift, 365–70. Amsterdam: Elsevier.

Wolfe, Patrick. 2006. "Settler Colonialism and the Elimination of the Native." *Journal of Genocide Research* 8, no. 4: 387–409. https://doi.org/10.1080/1462 3520601056240.

LEGAL RESOURCES

Indian Health Care Improvement Act, § 10221 of the Patient Protection and Affordable Care Act, Pub. L. No. 111–148, 124 Stat. 119 (2010)

Rosebud Sioux Tribe v. United States, 9 F.4th 1018 (8th Cir.) (2021)

Snyder Act, Pub. L. No. 67–85, 42 Stat. 208 (1921)

Treaty of Fort Laramie, Apr. 29, 1868, 15 T.S. 635 (1868)

PART I

HEALTH DISPARITIES IN INDIGENOUS COMMUNITIES

MARIANNE O. NIELSEN
AND KAREN JARRATT-SNIDER

S STATED IN THE INTRODUCTION, "health is a fundamental human right" according to the World Health Organization (WHO) (Ghebreyesus 2017). This means that governments are obligated by law to "ensure access to timely, acceptable, and affordable health care" of appropriate quality as well as providing for the underlying determinants of health such as "safe housing, water and sanitation" (WHO 2022). The WHO also declares that the needs of "those furthest behind" must be given priority, that this basic human right "must be enjoyed without discrimination on the grounds of race, age, ethnicity or any other factor" and that the people affected must have the right to participate in all aspects of service development and delivery (2022). There is little doubt that settler-colonial governments have failed miserably in living up to such legal and hence health obligations to their Indigenous Peoples. For example, a 2022 report by the U.S. Department of Health and Human Services (HHS) about health disparities among American Indian and Alaska Native populations notes, "Issues related to economic and social conditions in tribal communities are rooted in historical mistreatment of Native people in the U.S., such as forced relocation from tribal homelands to isolated areas, lack of funding for health-care services and infrastructure, and limited access to economic opportunities and other resources that affect social mobility" (HHS 2022, 2).

The report also notes the chronic and persistent underfunding of the Indian Health Service. Moreover, the leading cause of death for American Indians and Alaska Natives in 2020 was COVID-19, where the morbidity rate was 1.8 times higher than that for whites. Some other significant health disparities described by the report include that, compared to the overall U.S. population, American Indians and Alaska Natives have a 100 percent greater morbidity rate from homicide, a 64 percent greater morbidity rate of suicide, a 207 percent greater morbidity rate of diabetes mellitus, and a 133 percent greater morbidity rate from unintentional injuries (HHS 2022, 4). Clearly, the United States is falling short of ensuring that the fundamental human right of health is being met for Indigenous persons. Globally, it is not alone.

Not surprisingly, the United Nations (UN DESA 2016, 3) has argued that health care for the 370 million Indigenous people that live in ninety different countries is of major concern:

> Indigenous peoples face a myriad of obstacles when accessing public health systems. These include the lack of health facilities in indigenous communities and cultural differences with the health care providers such as differences in languages, illiteracy and lack of understanding of indigenous culture and traditional health care systems. There is also an absence of adequate health insurance or lack of economic capacity to pay for services. As a result, indigenous peoples often cannot afford health services even if [they are] available. Marginalization also means that indigenous peoples are reluctant or have difficulties in participating in non-indigenous processes or systems at the community, municipal, state and national levels.

The chapters in this section put this basic right of Indigenous individuals and nations into the broadest possible perspective by discussing the health of Indigenous inmates in the American criminal justice system, Indigenous veterans (Paquin), and the federal government's role in preserving Indigenous health (or not). Chapter 1, by Camplain et al., is one of the few scholarly documents that provides an overview of an often neglected population of Indigenous individuals—those incarcerated short-term in jails. Yet, as was discovered during the COVID pandemic, jails are breeding grounds for the spread of disease because of inadequate staffing and facilities. Conducting research with incarcerated Indigenous individuals is difficult. Correctional institutions are notoriously reluctant to allow researchers access to their populations—some of this reluctance is well intentioned, in order to protect this "captive population" from being subjected to research from which they receive little benefit, but some is not so well-intentioned and access is prohibited in order to protect the correctional institution itself. As Camplain et al. mention, cultural resources, which have a strong relation to mental well-being, are still not available to many incarcerated Indigenous individuals, whereas they are more readily available to non-Indigenous prisoners (see also Archambeault 2009). Physical health care is just as problematic, as Camplain et al. describe.

Paquin, in chapter 3, focuses on the special challenges faced by Indigenous veterans and their resilience in responding to them. Paquin's chapter offers a significant contribution to the sparse existing literature on the health and well-being of Native American veterans. Other works about Native American veterans do not focus exclusively on health and well-being (see, for example, Holm 1996; NMAI 2020).

In chapter 2, Dietrich and Schroedel trace the history of the American federal government's legal obligations to the Indigenous nations who ceded land. In turn, the federal government was obligated to provide a variety of services to protect the interests of American Indians and Alaska Natives, including housing, education, and most importantly for this book, health care. Not all treaties and agreements covered all the same health-care obligations on the part of the federal government. However, the right to health care for Indigenous individuals was enshrined in the federal government's fiduciary responsibilities and international declarations and covenants to which the United States was a signatory. The UN General Assembly's Universal Declaration of Human Rights (1948), for example, refers to "better standards of life" and states in Article 25.1, "Everyone has the right to a standard of living adequate for the health and well-being of himself and of his family, including food, clothing, housing *and medical care* and necessary social services, and the right to security in the event of unemployment, *sickness, disability,* widowhood, old age or other lack of livelihood in circumstances beyond his control" (UNGA 1948) (emphasis added). As Dietrich and Schroedel describe, the Indian Health Service has been and still is seriously remiss in helping the United States fulfill these obligations to its Indigenous Peoples.

The United States, instead of being a leader in providing health services to Indigenous Peoples, is yet another settler-colonial society that has failed its Indigenous Peoples in this area.

REFERENCES

Archambeault, William G. 2009. "The Search for the *Silver Arrow*: Assessing Tribal-Based Healing Traditions and Ceremonies in Indian Country Corrections." In *Criminal Justice in Native America*, edited by Marianne O. Nielsen and Robert A. Silverman, 191–206. Tucson: University of Arizona Press.

Ghebreyesus, Tedros Adhanom. 2017. "Health Is a Fundamental Human Right." World Health Organization. Commentary. December 10, 2017. https://www.who.int/news-room/commentaries/detail/health-is-a-fundamental-human-right.

HHS (U.S. Department of Health and Human Services). 2022. *How Increased Funding Can Advance the Mission of the Indian Health Service to Improve Health Outcomes for American Indians/Alaska Natives.* Report No. HP-2022–21. Washington, D.C.: Office of the Assistant Secretary for Planning and Evaluation, July 2022. https://aspe.hhs.gov/reports/funding-ihs.

Holm, Tom. 1996. *Strong Hearts, Wounded Souls: Native American Veterans of the Vietnam War.* Austin: University of Texas Press.

NMAI (National Museum of the American Indian). 2020. *Why We Serve: Native Americans in the United States Armed Forces.* Washington, D.C.: Smithsonian Books.

UN DESA (United Nations Department of Economic and Social Affairs). 2016. *State of the World's Indigenous Peoples: Indigenous Peoples'*

Access to Health Services. https://www.un.org/development/desa/indi
genouspeoples/wp-content/uploads/sites/19/2018/03/The-State-of
-The-Worlds-Indigenous-Peoples-WEB.pdf.

UNGA (United Nations General Assembly). 1948. Resolution 217A,
Universal Declaration of Human Rights. https://www.un.org/en
/about-us/universal-declaration-of-human-rights.

WHO (World Health Organization). 2022. "Human Rights." December 10, 2022. https://www.who.int/news-room/fact-sheets/detail
/human-rights-and-health.

LEGAL RESOURCES

United Nations Universal Declaration of Human Rights (1948)

1

INDIGENOUS PEOPLES' INVOLVEMENT IN THE U.S. JUSTICE SYSTEM, TRENDS, HEALTH IMPACTS, AND HEALTH DISPARITIES

RICKY CAMPLAIN, CARMENLITA CHIEF, CAROLYN CAMPLAIN, NICOLETTE I. TEUFEL-SHONE, AND JULIE BALDWIN

IT IS NOT NEW KNOWLEDGE that due to social, political, and economic factors, the United States has experienced an unmatched epidemic of criminal justice involvement compared to the rest of the world. Although the United States represents less than 5 percent of the world's population, of the more than 10.7 million people held in correctional institutions throughout the world, almost 20 percent are in the United States (Walmsley 2018). Fundamental explanations for the epidemic of incarceration are reflected in significant racial/ethnic disparities in criminal justice involvement. Over 60 percent of incarcerated populations are ethnic and racial minorities, although they make up just 30 percent of the U.S. population (Binswanger et al. 2012).

The burden of criminal justice involvement in the United States disproportionately affects communities of color, particularly Indigenous communities, compounding preexisting barriers to achieving health equity. Compared with the general population, incarcerated individuals have a higher burden of chronic diseases, including hypertension, diabetes, chronic respiratory conditions, and liver disease (Binswanger, Krueger, and Steiner 2009); communicable diseases, including hepatitis C, HIV, tuberculosis, and COVID-19 (Niveau 2006; Yang and Thompson 2020); and mental and behavioral health problems (Fazel and Danesh 2002).

The exposure to the physical environment of jails, including short-term stays and complicated by frequent re-incarcerations, creates short-term exposures to infectious diseases, interruption in the continuity of care for chronic diseases and behavioral health conditions, and potential barriers to prevention and treatment of substance use disorders. The exposure to prisons, long-term facilities in which individuals who are sentenced for a crime serve one year or longer, may cause longer-term impacts on health.

We understand the complicated nature of criminal justice involvement in the United States and how it impacts the health and well-being of individuals. In this chapter, we will discuss the unique challenges and complicated jurisdictions Indigenous populations face in the U.S. criminal justice system; trends in arrests, incarceration, and reentry; health disparities among incarcerated Indigenous populations; and promising practices and programs, including spiritual practices, for Indigenous people who are incarcerated.

UNDERSTANDING THE COMPLICATED JURISDICTIONS IN THE CRIMINAL JUSTICE SYSTEM FOR INDIGENOUS POPULATIONS IN THE UNITED STATES

The U.S. criminal justice system is an organization that exists to enforce legal codes. There are three branches that include the police, the courts, and the corrections system (e.g., jails and prisons). However, to categorize the U.S. criminal justice system into three groups is a vast simplification. There is entry into the system, which includes police interactions and arrests; prosecution and pretrial services; adjudication; sentencing and sanctions; and corrections (jails and prisons) (BJS 2021). However, the figure below provides a simplified view of the case flow throughout the criminal justice system.

The corrections system in particular is made up of jails and prisons. The majority of prisons are correctional facilities, run by the state or federal government, that hold individuals with sentences longer than one year, whereas jails generally are short-term correctional facilities, run by local law enforcement (counties, cities, towns) or government agencies including tribal law enforcement, designed to hold individuals awaiting trial or serving sentences of less than one year (BJS 2018).

What is the sequence of events in the criminal justice system?

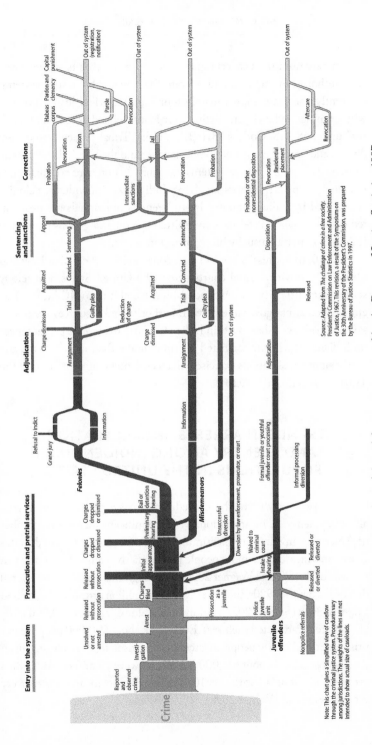

Note: This chart gives a simplified view of caseflow through the criminal justice system. Procedures vary among jurisdictions. The weights of the lines are not intended to show actual size of caseloads.

Source: Adapted from *The challenge of crime in a free society.* President's Commission on Law Enforcement and Administration of Justice, 1967. This revision, a result of the Symposium on the 30th Anniversary of the President's Commission, was prepared by the Bureau of Justice Statistics in 1997.

FIGURE 1.1 Criminal Justice System Flowchart. Adapted from a report revised by the Bureau of Justice Statistics, 1997.

Separate from the U.S. criminal justice system, tribes have the sovereign authority to establish and operate their own tribal justice systems. Currently, there are approximately four hundred tribal justice systems with criminal and civil jurisdiction over lands defined as "Indian Country" under 18 U.S. Code § 1511 (BIA, n.d.). Tribal justice systems are diverse and unique compared to one another and the U.S. judicial system. In most cases, tribal justice systems have jurisdiction over criminal cases that include misdemeanors involving Indigenous individuals. Felonies committed in Indian Country by Indigenous individuals are heard in federal court, whereas felonies committed by non-Indigenous persons in Indian Country are usually brought to state court.

In 2010, to address crime in tribal communities, the Tribal Law and Order Act provided tribal courts across the United States new felony sentencing authority and expanded punitive abilities (NCAI, n.d.). It empowered tribal governments with authority and resources for public safety and allows tribal courts in Indian Country to increase jail sentences for individuals who are convicted of crimes under their jurisdiction. Currently, eight tribal nations exercise enhanced sentencing provisions of the Tribal Law and Order Act.

TRENDS IN ARRESTS, INCARCERATION, AND REENTRY AMONG INDIGENOUS POPULATIONS IN THE UNITED STATES

Over the past forty years, the United States has experienced an unparalleled epidemic of incarceration, with a significant increase in number of Americans involved in the criminal justice system. The United States arrests and incarcerates more people per capita than any other country in the world (Sawyer and Wagner 2020). Although there has been an overall decrease from the 1990s, there were over 10.1 million arrests in the United States in 2019 (Statista 2022). Additionally, almost 700 per 100,000 individuals are incarcerated each year. Every year, about 600,000 people enter prison, with 1,291,000 people incarcerated in prison in total. On any given day, local jails hold about 631,000 people. However, 9 million Americans cycle in and out of jail, with over 10.6 million distinct incarcerations every year (Sawyer and Wagner 2020).

People of color are disproportionately represented in the U.S. criminal justice system (Mauer and King 2007). Over 60 percent of incarcerated populations are ethnic/racial minorities even though those groups make up just 30 percent of the U.S. population (Morgan et al. 2014; Binswanger et al. 2012; Bai et al. 2015). Black and Latino men have a 1-in-3 and 1-in-6 lifetime risk of incarceration, respectively, compared to a 1-in-23 lifetime risk among non-Hispanic white men (Bonczar 2003). Additionally, racial/ethnic minority individuals are more likely to be charged or fully prosecuted compared to their white counterparts (Wu 2016). However, the overrepresentation of Indigenous people in the U.S. criminal justice system has been overlooked. Indigenous people have an incarceration rate of 1,291 per 100,000, almost double that of the national rate and over double that of white Americans (510 per 100,000) (Daniel 2020). In states with larger Indigenous populations, the incarceration rates can be over seven times that of whites. Unfortunately, information and data regarding Indigenous individuals incarcerated in the United States are scarce.

In other countries, the data is clearer regarding Indigenous people who are incarcerated. In Canada, there is an extreme overrepresentation of Indigenous people in prisons and jails. Indigenous people represent about 4.1 percent of the Canadian population but 28 percent of the incarcerated population. Indigenous women make up 40 percent of women who are incarcerated. From 2009 to 2018, the incarcerated population increased by less than 1 percent while the Indigenous incarceration rate rose by 42.8 percent. Overall, the rate of incarceration of Indigenous men is over eight times higher than that of non-Indigenous men; the rate of incarceration of Indigenous women is 12.5 times that of non-Indigenous women (Department of Justice Canada 2023). Aboriginal and Torres Strait Islanders (Indigenous Peoples of Australia) show similar rates: they make up about 3.2 percent of the Australian population while making up 32 percent of all individuals who are incarcerated (Australian Bureau of Statistics 2022, 2023).

ARRESTS

There is a long-standing history of disparities in arrests among Indigenous people: Indigenous people have a higher arrest risk in the United

States than any other racial/ethnic group (Barnes et al. 2015). Indigenous people in 1960 were arrested at a rate of 15,123 per 100,000, compared to 5,908 for African Americans and 1,655 for whites (Lester 1999). More recently, despite making up only 9 percent of Flagstaff, Arizona, residents, Indigenous people make up 45 percent of Flagstaff Police Department arrests (J. Brown 2014). In Montana, Indigenous people make up 7 percent of the population but account for about 20 percent of arrests (CSG Justice Center 2015). Additionally, Indigenous women comprise 1.4 percent of the population of women in Minneapolis, Minnesota, but make up 6.6 percent of police stops (Gorsuch and Rho 2019). After they were stopped, 27 percent and 20 percent of Indigenous women were searched and booked into jail, respectively, compared to 6 percent and 4 percent of white women.

Police arrest Indigenous people for violent and property crimes at twice the rate of the greater U.S. population (Tighe 2014). Indigenous people are more likely than their white counterparts to be arrested for murder, aggravated assault, and motor vehicle theft and less likely to be arrested for weapon-law violations and drug possession and sales (Snyder 2011). In the United States, the arrest rate among Indigenous people for all alcohol violations (driving under the influence, violating liquor laws, public intoxication) was more than double that of the total population, at 2,545 per 100,000 compared to 1,079 per 100,000 overall (Steele, Damon, and Denman 2004). More specifically, Indigenous people were arrested for driving under the influence at a rate of 479 per 100,000, compared to 332 per 100,000 overall, and arrested for liquor law violations at a rate of 405 per 100,000, compared to 143 per 100,000 overall (Perry 2004).

Although Indigenous people are arrested at a higher rate, there is evidence that this is not due to Indigenous people committing more crimes. Police interactions with racial/ethnic minorities, including Indigenous people, are more likely to result in arrest compared to interactions with white individuals (Kochel, Wilson, and Mastrofski 2011). The higher arrest rate persists even after accounting for decision-making by police. Furthermore, racial/ethnic minorities are more likely to experience negative consequences, such as arrest and detainment, due to racial discrimination and stigmas (Mulia et al. 2008). For example, Indigenous people have a history of overrepresentation in the criminal justice system for alcohol-related offenses, particularly in the Southwest (Feldstein, Venner, and

May 2006). However, Indigenous people in the Southwest have higher alcohol abstention rates compared to the general U.S. population (Spicer et al. 2003).

In addition, the firewater myth—the idea that Indigenous people in the United States have biological or genetic differences that make them more prone to the impact of alcohol and are more at risk for alcohol-related issues (Gonzalez and Skewes 2016)—is a rampant stereotype pushed by inaccurate history and the media. In reality, according to a study done by Cunningham Solomon, and Muramoto (2016) using the National Survey on Drug Use and Health and the Behavioral Risk Factor Surveillance System, almost 60 percent of Indigenous people abstained from alcohol in the month before the survey, compared to only about 43 percent of white Americans. The study also found that there was no significant difference between white and Indigenous binge drinkers or heavy drinkers in either survey.

INCARCERATION

A higher proportion of police interactions with Indigenous individuals not only lead to an arrest but also lead to a booking into a local jail facility, compared to the general U.S. population and other racial/ethnic groups (Camplain et al. 2020). Between 1999 and 2014, the number of Indigenous people in local jails increased by 90 percent, while the percentage of white individuals incarcerated in local jails stayed about the same (Minton and Cowhig 2020). According to the Bureau of Justice Statistics (BJS), Indigenous people are incarcerated at a rate that is 38 percent higher than the national average (Greenfeld and Smith 1999). For example, in one southwestern county, Indigenous people were more likely than white, Latine, and Black people to be booked into jail, rather than cited and released at time of arrest for misdemeanor drug- and alcohol-related charges. Furthermore, Indigenous people had higher odds of being convicted and serving time for their misdemeanor and felony drug- and alcohol-related arrests than their white, Latine, and Black counterparts (Camplain et al. 2020). Notably, although 90 percent of Indigenous individuals arrested in the United States were sentenced to imprisonment, almost half of Indigenous individuals arrested had little or no prior criminal history (U.S. Sentencing Commission 2013). These types of disparities

TABLE 1.1 Percent of Indigenous People in a State's Population Compared to Percent Incarcerated in Jail and Prison in States with High Proportion of Indigenous People

STATE	PERCENT OF INDIGENOUS PEOPLE IN THE POPULATION	PERCENT OF INDIGENOUS PEOPLE INCARCERATED
Alaska	15	38
Arizona	5	10
Minnesota	1	8
Montana	6	22
New Mexico	9	11
North Dakota	5	29
Oklahoma	7	8
South Dakota	9	29
Utah	1	4
Washington	2	5

Source: Jones (2018)

lead to extremely high rates of Indigenous individuals incarcerated in jail and prisons compared to other racial/ethnic groups.

In 2010, there were a total of 37,854 Indigenous people (American Indians and Alaskan Natives) in adult correctional facilities (not including tribal jails), including 32,524 men and 5,132 women (and 198 people who were under the age of eighteen) (Daniel 2020). However, similar to arrests, in states with large Indigenous populations, such as North Dakota and Montana, Indigenous incarceration rates can be up to seven times that of whites. Other states with large Indigenous populations, including Alaska, Arizona, Minnesota, New Mexico, Oklahoma, South Dakota, Utah, and Washington, have higher proportions of Indigenous individuals incarcerated (Jones 2018). For example, Indigenous people are about four times more likely to be incarcerated than whites in Arizona. From 1999 to 2014, the percentage of Indigenous people in Arizona jails more than doubled—the largest increase in any state (Minton and Cowhig 2020).

An estimated 9,700 Indigenous people (401 per 100,000 population) were incarcerated in local jails, facilities that individuals are typically booked into when arrested and that house individuals awaiting adjudication or serving sentences of less than a year (Zeng 2018). That is twice the jail incarceration rates for both white and Latine people (187 and 185 per 100,000, respectively). In one southwestern county, Indigenous

TABLE 1.2 Percent of Indigenous People in a State's Population Compared to Percent Incarcerated in Prison in States with High Proportion of Indigenous People

STATE	NUMBER OF INDIGENOUS PEOPLE INCARCERATED IN PRISON	PERCENT OF INDIGENOUS PEOPLE INCARCERATED IN PRISON	PERCENT OF INDIGENOUS PEOPLE IN THE POPULATION
Alaska	1,611	36	15
Arizona	2,281	5	5
Colorado	666	3	1
Minnesota	1,046	10	1
Montana	817	22	6
New Mexico	500	7	9
North Carolina	946	3	1
North Dakota	342	20	5
Oklahoma	3,133	11	7
South Dakota	1,301	33	9
Utah	310	5	1
Washington	934	5	2
Wisconsin	900	4	1

Source: Bronson and Carson (2019)

people make up 33 percent of all incarcerations over a seventeen-year period. Additionally, 61 percent of Indigenous men and 51 percent of Indigenous women were incarcerated more than once, the highest of any gender/racial/ethnic group in the county (40 percent overall). Further, 9.2 percent and 4.7 percent of Indigenous men and women, respectively, were incarcerated more than ten times, compared to 3.7 percent of the aggregate sample (Camplain, Warren, et al. 2019).

Tribal jails, or jails in Indian Country, are "adult and juvenile detention centers, jails, and other correctional facilities operated by tribal authorities or the Bureau of Indian Affairs" (BJS, n.d.). Little is known regarding incarceration in the eighty-four tribal jails in the United States. In those jails, an estimated 9,360 people were admitted in June 2018, with 2,870 individuals incarcerated at midyear (one point in time), an increase from about 2,000 in 2010 (Minton and Cowhig 2020). In general, tribal jails hold about 2,500–2,820 people daily (Sawyer and Wagner 2020; Minton and Cowhig 2020); however, from aforementioned general jail statistics, it is clear that represents only a fraction of incarcerated Indigenous persons.

In 2017, 23,701 Indigenous people were incarcerated in prison, long-term facilities housing individuals convicted of a crime and serving sentences greater than or equal to one year (about 1.6 percent of all individuals incarcerated in U.S. prisons) (Bronson and Carson 2019). This was an increase from 19,790 Indigenous men and 2,954 Indigenous women incarcerated in state and federal prisons in 2016. From 2008 to 2013, the number of Indigenous Americans incarcerated in federal prisons has increased by 27 percent (U.S. Sentencing Commission 2013). In nineteen U.S. states, Indigenous populations are more overrepresented in the prison population than any other racial/ethnic group (Sakala 2014). States including Alaska, Minnesota, Montana, North Dakota, Oklahoma, and South Dakota, have notably high proportions of Indigenous people incarcerated in prisons (Bronson and Carson 2019).

REENTRY

Indigenous women and men are reincarcerated faster and more often compared to other racial/ethnic groups. Upon release into the community from prison, 45 percent of Indigenous individuals returned to prison within thirty-six months (Washington State Department of Corrections 2020); another study showed that 36 percent of Indigenous people released from prison were reincarcerated for a technical violation of their probation or parole (Perry 2004), about three times the rate for whites (Hartney and Vuong 2009). Almost half of Indigenous people released from prison in 1994 were convicted of a new crime within three years (Perry 2004). About 21 percent of those individuals were sentenced to prison for the new offense(s). Indigenous people are over twice as likely as others to return to an institution in Montana, for instance, regardless of gender, age, education, criminal history, or mental health (Conley and Schantz 2006).

In addition to higher rates of incarceration and reincarceration, Indigenous people are put on parole at twice the rate of whites (Hartney and Vuong 2009). More specifically, Indigenous people had higher parole rates than those for whites in the District of Columbia and twenty-six states with over five times the rates for whites in Iowa, Minnesota, Nebraska, New York, and Wisconsin (Hartney and Vuong 2009).

HEALTH DISPARITIES AMONG INDIGENOUS PEOPLE INVOLVED THE U.S. JUSTICE SYSTEM

It is not new information that, compared with the general population, individuals involved in the criminal justice system, particularly those who are incarcerated, have a higher burden of chronic diseases, communicable diseases, and mental and behavioral health disorders (Binswanger, Krueger, and Steiner 2009; Niveau 2006; Maruschak, Berzofsky, and Unangst 2015; Fazel and Danesh 2002). In 2011–12, about 40 percent of individuals incarcerated in prison and jail self-reported having a chronic medical condition, with high blood pressure being the most common chronic condition (26–30 percent). Additionally, 14 percent reported having tuberculosis, hepatitis B or C, or a sexually transmitted infection (Maruschak, Berzofsky, and Unangst 2015).

We would be remiss if we did not mention that there are many factors in the correctional environment that may contribute to health disparities among incarcerated individuals, along with many additional factors that impact the health and well-being of Indigenous people specifically. For example, diabetes and cardiovascular disease are managed through behavior, particularly food choices and exercise, and/or medication. Dietary recommendations include intake of low-fat and high-fiber foods, and activity recommendations include a minimum of thirty minutes of moderate activity five days a week. Incarcerated individuals have limited autonomy over the types of foods they can eat and the amount of physical activity in which they can participate (Camplain, Baldwin, et al. 2019; Camplain et al. 2022). Thus, behavioral management of diabetes, cardiovascular disease, and their risk factors such as high blood pressure can be difficult in a restrictive environment; this may contribute to increased severity of symptoms and side effects and even advancement of secondary complications, such as renal disease, retinopathy, and stroke. Further, access to health care may be limited while people are incarcerated and discontinued and hindered after release. Although health care is a constitutional right to individuals who are incarcerated, people in prisons and jails often face limited, inadequate, and, occasionally, no access to medical care, examinations, and prescription medication (Wilper et al. 2009). Once released, continuity of care is further hindered by distrust, discrimination, poor communication, and racism in the health-care system (Puglisi, Calderon, and Wang 2017).

Non-institutionalized Indigenous people suffer from many health disparities, often due to structural and interpersonal racism, barriers to health-care access, and historical trauma. Indigenous people have long experienced lower health status compared with other racial/ethnic groups, including lower life expectancy and disproportionate disease burden (Jones 2006; Hutchinson and Shin 2014). Indigenous people have a life expectancy 5.5 years less than the U.S. population as a whole. Furthermore, Indigenous people suffer from cardiovascular disease and associated factors, including obesity, metabolic syndrome, hypertension, hyperlipidemia, and diabetes at a higher rate than other racial/ethnic groups and the general U.S. population (Hutchinson and Shin 2014). Additionally, early-onset diabetes impacts Indigenous populations more often than other racial/ethnic groups (Moore 2010). This is impactful, because the majority of individuals that interact with the criminal justice system are younger than forty-five years. Indigenous people are more likely to also have certain cancers such as liver, stomach, lung, colorectal, and kidney cancers (Wiggins et al. 2008). Finally, Indigenous populations disproportionately suffer from mental health problems including anxiety, depression, substance use disorders, post-traumatic stress disorder, and suicide, due to associated risk factors such as poverty, historical trauma, victimization, lack of health insurance, and lack of access to appropriate health care (HHS 2001; Beals et al. 2005; Gone and Trimble 2012).

There is ample evidence that Indigenous people in the general population suffer from poorer health compared to other racial/ethnic groups; thus, it is reasonable to conclude that Indigenous people that are impacted by the criminal justice system are also experiencing poorer health than their non-Native counterparts. However, little research exists on the health of Indigenous people who are incarcerated and what little research has been done either aggregates data for all racial/ethnic groups or classifies Indigenous people into an "other" group due to small or insufficient sample size (Bai et al. 2015).

Among a sample of individuals incarcerated in a jail whose population was composed of almost 60 percent Indigenous people, over 25 percent reported having fair or poor general health, an independent predictor of cardiovascular and all-cause mortality (Barger, Cribbet, and Muldoon

2016). A high proportion of all individuals incarcerated in this south-western county jail also reported being overweight or obese (61 percent) and/or having hypertension (36 percent), high cholesterol (18 percent), arthritis (18 percent), asthma (15 percent), diabetes (12 percent), a liver condition (12 percent), hepatitis C (7 percent), HIV (5 percent), hepatitis B (3 percent), and/or tuberculosis (2 percent) (Trotter, Lininger, et al. 2018). In addition to chronic and/or communicable medical conditions, a high proportion of individuals reported having anxiety (37 percent), depression (34 percent), post-traumatic stress disorder (26 percent), ADD/ADHD (23 percent), bipolar disorder (20 percent), and/or schizophrenia (11 percent) (Trotter, Lininger, et al. 2018).

PROMISING PRACTICES AND PROGRAMS IN JAILS AND PRISONS, AND FOR REENTRY AMONG INDIGENOUS PEOPLE INVOLVED IN THE U.S. JUSTICE SYSTEM

To more fully grasp the significance of strides made in recent decades to introduce Indigenous cultural and spiritual practices into correctional facilities, these practices must be understood within the context of colonialism. The Indigenous experience with settler-colonial states through systemic means of oppression is a long one. Countries such as the United States, Canada, and Australia have historically passed and upheld national and state or provincial laws aimed at dismantling Indigenous cultural identities and traditions through religious suppression—instituting bans on practices and rites expressive of Indigenous spirituality, obstructing access to sacred sites, and outlawing possession of ceremonial objects such as peyote and sacred pipes (Irwin 2006).

Attempting to simplify Indigenous religious beliefs and practices for generalizable consumption is a daunting and nearly impossible task. Generally, most Indigenous Peoples around the world view their everyday cultural ways of being and living as being spiritually purposeful and significant. Hence, culture and spirituality (or religious practice) are inextricably connected because one structures the other. Unlike Euro-Western notions of religion, which impose a separation between God and the world we exist in, Indigenous spirituality and religious orientations see a

Creator or multiple sacred deities as a part of the world. This difference in the perception of religion and the human relationship to the "holy" is but one aspect of the Othering process employed by Westerners to cast Indigenous Peoples as primitive, ahistorical, unsophisticated, uncivilized, unstable, and savage nonhumans. This was a means to justify colonial tactics of genocide (e.g., subjugation of Indigenous Peoples, atrocious acts of violence, removal from homelands, and cultural assimilation) that were employed in order to lay claim to Indigenous land and natural resources for the establishment of settler-colonial expansion, wealth, and prosperity (Nielsen and Robyn 2019).

Indigenous individuals have only been granted U.S. citizenship within the last century through the Indian Citizenship Act of 1924, which also conferred the right to vote. After that, it took another half century before all Native citizens were afforded protection of the right to practice their religious, spiritual, and cultural beliefs, with the 1978 passage of the American Indian Religious Freedom Act (AIRFA). Between 1993 and 2000, the Religious Freedom Restoration Act (RFRA) and the Religious Land Use and Institutionalized Persons Act (RLUIPA) were passed to increase these protections. Regarding RFRA and RLUIPA, a guidance document produced by the Native American Rights Fund (2016) and intended for Indigenous people in correctional facilities explains, "Both statutes prevent the government from substantially burdening [an inmate's] religious practice unless it has a compelling reason to do so in [the inmate's] particular case," and that prisons may only burden or hinder religious practices if they have "no other, less restrictive alternatives available." Admittedly, this is a very condensed presentation of some of the historical strides made by the U.S. government to suppress and then protect and preserve Indigenous traditional religious beliefs and practices, but this contextual information is pertinent for understanding the advances made from the 1960s forward.

The 1960s and 1970s marked a social movement in the United States that was pushing for the right of Indigenous individuals who were incarcerated to exercise their Native religious practices. In the early 1960s, Clyde Bellecourt, an Anishinaabe (Ojibwe) man, met a young Anishinaabe spiritual leader named Eddie Benton-Banai when they were both serving time in Minnesota's Stillwater prison (Reha 2001). Bellecourt and Benton-Banai, known for their founding roles in the American Indian

Movement, formed the American Indian Folklore Group while incarcerated, to help incarcerated Indigenous people heal by learning about Native history, epistemologies, culture, and spirituality through pan-Indian frameworks (Tighe 2014). Tighe (2014, 5) describes this effort as a "model for Indian cultural renaissance within prisons." Bellecourt affirms that ceremonies are an integral component of the healing process that can support individuals involved in the criminal justice system to make positive changes in their lives, and credits how establishing a spiritual base in his own life helped him to overcome his battle with alcoholism (Reha 2001).

With the aid of the Native American Rights Fund, one of the oldest and largest legal organizations committed to defending the legal rights of Indigenous people and nations, Indigenous individuals incarcerated in Nebraska won a federal court consent decree in *Wolff v. McDonnell* (1974), which allowed them to practice their religious and cultural beliefs in prison. This opened the way in Nebraska for sweat lodges to be conducted, Native clubs and spiritual collectives to be formed, and elders to serve as spiritual advisors and cultural-based counselors inside correctional facilities (Irwin 2006). Irwin (2006, 42) notes that the consent decree "established an important precedent for native prisoners in other states."

Traction on this issue continued to grow in other parts of the United States during the late 1970s and early 1980s. Incarcerated Indigenous people were increasingly bringing suits against prison administrators for denying their rights to religious freedom. In the Southwest, the Navajo Nation appointed a Navajo spiritual advisor who eventually was conducting ceremonies in nineteen prisons throughout the region (Echo-Hawk 1996). Incarcerated Indigenous women formed a spiritual organization within a Montana state prison in the early 1990s and perceived their unification as threatening to prison staff (Ross 1998). As a way of weakening the close bonds formed through the organization, the women felt staff strategically targeted Indigenous women who were labeled as "troublemakers" and then written up for "trumped-up charges" (Ross 1998, 243) which resulted in their transfer to a maximum-security facility. White women incarcerated in prison interviewed by Ross also noticed the same pattern, identifying it as "prejudiced" practice (265). At that time, Indigenous women made up 25 percent of the prison population while making up 6 percent of the Montana state population. In addition to the institutional discrimination experienced by incarcerated Indigenous women,

Ross (278) notes the direct racist remarks about "Indians" and "Indian culture" made by prison staff and incarcerated white individuals to her and incarcerated Indigenous individual. By the time RFRA was passed in 1993, a large number of successful suits were being filed by Indigenous individuals incarcerated in prison, who were protesting infringement of their religious and spiritual needs and advocating for the right to bring traditional tobacco pipe and sweat lodge ceremonies into the prison complex (Irwin 2006).

SPIRITUAL PRACTICES IN JAILS AND PRISONS—WHAT DO THEY LOOK LIKE NOW? WHAT NEEDS TO BE DONE?

Many incarcerated individuals do not have deep awareness of their Indigenous culture or languages due to family or cultural distancing linked to direct or intergenerational trauma from their experiences in boarding schools and foster care and adoption programs (Waldram 2020). Pipe and sweat lodge ceremonies, or "sweats" as they are also called, have long been vital traditions and healing practices for many Indigenous individuals, Peoples, and nations (Irwin 2006). Though protocols for participation in these ceremonies may differ by nation or region, Indigenous Peoples hold in common the understanding that ceremonies provide an avenue for purification and cleansing of the body, mind, and spirit and, thus, healing and restoration of harmony (Irwin 2006). In alignment with Indigenous world views regarding the importance of community support, kinship, and relationships, these ceremonies are conducted as a group in the presence of an individual's support network, such as family, extended relatives, and fellow community members (Irwin 2006; Echo-Hawk 1996). According to advocates such as Archie Fire Lame Deer, a Lakota spiritual leader and substance abuse counselor who was instrumental in bringing Lakota purification ceremonies into California prisons during the 1970s, the sweat lodge ceremony holds enormous redemptive value, as it helps Indigenous incarcerated individuals to evaluate their conduct by reframing and restoring the relationships they have with others inside and outside of the prison complex, which lends to their general sense of well-being (Irwin 2006).

Irwin (2006) reports that up to 65 percent of incarcerated Indigenous individuals experience sweat and pipe ceremonies for the first time in prison, and this introduction provides a means for developing a stronger sense of Indigenous identity and cooperation with other incarcerated Indigenous individuals from a wide diversity of Indigenous communities. Irwin also describes the use of pipe and sweat lodge ceremonies in correctional facilities as a new movement of pan-Native spirituality expressing intertribal unity, spiritual self-affirmation, and fostering respect for others, essentially building a path to peace and harmony both inside and outside of prison. Programs now being run in many reservation communities by formerly incarcerated individuals, as well as spiritual advisers, are continuing the "way of the pipe" in conjunction with the Red Road and the White Bison Wellbriety Movement approaches to substance abuse recovery (Wellbriety Circles 2021; Red Road 2021). These programs are offered in treatment facilities, halfway houses, and community prayer circles using the strategies that originated in prison (Irwin 2006; Ross 1998; Waldram 2020). A movement that began with alienated incarcerated Indigenous people has emerged as a source of healing and reintegration for not only this specific population but also for returning and non-incarcerated community members struggling with trauma and addiction.

Since the mid-2000s, spiritual practices and ceremonies have been implemented increasingly in correctional centers as a culturally based form of therapeutic healing, often used for anger management and substance abuse recovery (Garrett et al. 2011; Parks and Surowidjojo 2020; Irwin 2006). Examples from specific regions and correctional facilities documented in the peer-reviewed literature are sparse, yet stories do appear in the media, describing cultural and spiritual programs and ceremonies conducted in correctional facilities in California (Chaddock 2018), Maine (Casey 2020), New Mexico (Haywood 2019), Oklahoma (Brewer 2016), Oregon (Parks and Surowidjojo 2020), Utah (T. Brown 2014), and Washington (Hopper 2021). A comprehensive list of cultural and spiritual programs for Indigenous people incarcerated in the United States is not available, so the consistency and sustainability of the programs described in media is unknown.

An impact study conducted by Gossage et al. (2003) describes the Diné Center for Substance Abuse Treatment staff's use of sweat lodge ceremonies as a modality for jail-based, substance abuse recovery treatment with Indigenous men. In post-incarceration data collection with 190 men (ages eighteen to sixty-four years) who participated in ceremonies while imprisoned, most reported a reduction in the number of drinks consumed in drinking sessions. The paucity of research on the impact of these programs calls for an increase in effectiveness studies to determine if these interventions are acceptable, sustainable with current levels of facility funding, and cost effective.

Most incarcerated Indigenous individuals will return home. Blythe George (2020), a Yurok scholar, highlights Native nations' investment in reentry efforts. In the last decade, regional and national movements such as Native American Reentry Services have emerged to facilitate the transition from incarceration to home communities. These programs often work in correctional facilities to provide spiritual and cultural programs for Indigenous individuals to support self-reflection and to begin the healing and reorientation process. As a component of the federal government's trust responsibility to Native nations, funding should be provided to support partnerships between researchers and correctional facilities to assess the characteristics, feasibility, sustainability, impact, and cost effectiveness of these in-facility and transition programs. Given the high rate of incarceration among Indigenous people and the expense of incarceration and recidivism, identifying solutions to support Indigenous people to return to their communities and general society could contribute to national efforts to reduce mass incarceration and the unequal burden on populations of color (Echo-Hawk 1996; Blankenship et al. 2018; Bazelon 2020).

TRADITION AND RESILIENCE

Traditionally, Indigenous communities have favored a less adversarial approach to justice, emphasizing healing, resolution, and personal responsibility. The therapeutic jurisprudence model focuses on clients' well-being, addressing their psychological, spiritual, social, and emotional challenges and needs (Flies-Away, Gardner, and Carrow 2014). Under this model, lawyers and judges, in some cases in collaboration with social workers and mental health professionals, act as therapeutic agents working to minimize psychological harms endured by individuals who are charged with crimes and define a plan of action to reduce recidivism (Winick

2013). The approach uses an ethic of care, emphasizes self-determination (not paternalism), and employs motivational interviewing of individuals involved in the criminal justice system to explore strategies to reduce repeated criminal behaviors (Feldstein and Ginsburg 2006). Similarly, restorative justice, often combined with therapeutic jurisprudence, facilitates meetings between the victim(s) and the individual(s) charged with the crime to resolve collectively how to deal with the aftermath of the offense and its implication for the future; in some cases, the community is represented as a victim (Braithwaite 1999). The fundamental principle of restorative justice is that the crime is a violation of relationships rather than merely a violation of a law (Zehr 1990). Therapeutic jurisprudence and restorative justice are aligned with traditional Indigenous approaches to conflict resolution, victim healing, and the rehabilitation and reintegration of the individual charged with the crime into the community (Metoui 2007).

In 1997, the Office of Justice Programs of the U.S. Department of Justice launched the Tribal Healing to Wellness Courts program, which provides therapeutic jurisprudence training developed by the National Association of Drug Court Professionals and a Tribal Advisory Committee (Tribal Law and Policy Institute 2003). The U.S. Bureau of Justice Assistance provided competitive funding to support tribal courts to develop locally relevant procedures and court codes, and to apply this alternative approach. In 2003, the Tribal Law and Policy Institute prepared a monograph in collaboration with the Department of Justice to codify the key components (Flies-Away, Garrow, and Sekaquaptewa 2014). Since 2003, the Tribal Law and Policy Institute has developed multiple resources, e.g., treatment guidelines, case management guidance, policies and procedures, bench cards (resource materials for judges and court-appointed professionals), and updates on the key component monograph (BJA, n.d.). In 2010, ninety tribes either had an active wellness court or a wellness court at some time in past (Tribal Law and Policy Institute 2003). Evaluation of impact has been sporadic, and the programs have been difficult to sustain, with tribes citing lack of financial resources and limited time of court personnel and community members who serve as mentors. Evaluation with four tribal wellness courts showed programs have been more effective with adults than with juveniles, program graduates took longer to reoffend than did nongraduates, and participants reported reducing their alcohol and substance abuse (Gottlieb 2005). Participants, their families, and wellness court members (court personnel and community members) in these four communities described their wellness courts as successful. Participants appreciated the empathy of the counselors and mentors, and the tie to culture and traditional forms of justice, with several participants indicating they had turned their lives around. The 2005 evaluation report states that "people's subjective opinions of how the wellness court succeeded were more optimistic than the statistical recidivism rates" (Gottlieb 2005, ix–x).

CONCLUSIONS: LOOKING TO THE FUTURE

This chapter addresses the unique challenges Indigenous Peoples and individuals face in the U.S. criminal justice system; the oversight from multiple levels of government including federal, state, county, city, and tribal; trends in arrests, incarceration, and reentry; health disparities among Indigenous populations incarcerated in the United States; and promising practices and programs for Indigenous populations involved in the justice system.

As noted earlier, there are significant racial/ethnic disparities in criminal justice involvement. These disparities are also sharply evident in health outcomes. Empirical research demonstrates that compared to the general population, incarcerated individuals experience higher levels of chronic conditions (Bai et al. 2015), communicable diseases (Massoglia 2008), and poorer mental health outcomes (Fazel and Danesh 2002). Also, currently thirty-one states suspend or reclassify Medicaid for the duration of incarceration or for a specific amount of time, while the remaining nineteen states terminate Medicaid while the individual is incarcerated. This creates a barrier to continuity of care for many chronic conditions, treatment regimens for severe mental illness, and other behavioral health problems (Trotter, Camplain, et al. 2018; Trotter, Lininger, et al. 2018). There is ample evidence that Indigenous people in the general population suffer from poorer health than other racial/ethnic groups. Thus, it follows that Indigenous people who are impacted by the criminal justice system are also experiencing poorer health than their non-Indigenous counterparts.

Although there are apparent health disparities among incarcerated individuals, there is still little public health research being conducted among individuals involved in the criminal justice system, specifically those incarcerated in jails. We found research on health issues and incarceration, especially on jail versus prison incarceration, to be relatively scarce and predominantly single disease oriented. Extant research focuses overwhelmingly on relatively stable prison populations as opposed to the much more transient local jail populations (Binswanger, Krueger, and Steiner 2009; Massoglia 2008). To assess criminal and health-care history among individuals incarcerated, numerous sources of data have to be linked, including incarceration records, jail medical records, primary care patient records, and general information on access to health-care services.

We are addressing the primary social and environmental impacts on the health of incarcerated individuals by taking the position that a simple categorical approach (single disease, single solution) ultimately fails to appropriately address the public health ecology of incarceration and its impact on population health. Promising practices for Indigenous people in the U.S. justice system also emphasize the importance of understanding these practices against the backdrop of settler colonialism and the importance of introducing Indigenous cultural and spiritual practices into correctional facilities, as well as the importance of increased recognition of these practices by prison officials as legitimate religious needs that are integral for Indigenous healing. Several examples were shared in this chapter that have met with success. Between 1978 and 2000, AIRFA, RFRA, and RLUIPA were passed to afford and expand Indigenous protection of their right to practice their religious, spiritual, and cultural beliefs. A 2016 guidance document explains that both RFRA and RLUIPA prevent the government from hindering religious and spiritual practices of Indigenous people in correctional facilities. Advances and social movements since the 1960s have shown that Indigenous people who are incarcerated heal by learning about Indigenous history, epistemologies, culture, and spirituality. Ceremonies are an integral component of the healing process (Reha 2001). In addition to social movements, there were many Indigenous wins in the court system defending the legal rights of Indigenous Peoples, individuals, and nations.

Indigenous communities have traditionally taken a less adversarial and punitive approach to justice, instead focusing on healing, resolution, personal responsibility, and restoring relationships between the individual who committed the crime and those affected by offending actions. In this chapter, the therapeutic jurisprudence model and restorative justice approach are brought forward as frameworks that align with Indigenous values supportive of healthy conflict resolution, victim healing, and the rehabilitation and reintegration of the individual who committed the crime into the community. Since the late 1990s, tribal wellness court programs have emerged and increased in numbers with federal funding support. By 2010, approximately 90 Indigenous nations had a wellness court program, either currently or in the recent past. In 2014, it was reported that 120 Indigenous communities had implemented a Tribal Healing to Wellness court program, many of which were recently established (Tribal Law and Policy Institute 2017). Wellness court programs apply a teams-based, multisectoral approach, involving the community, to promote wellness as an ongoing journey for program participants, restoration and advancement of community well-being, and more broadly, promotion of Nation building and tribal sovereignty. An evaluation of four tribal wellness courts showed the programs to be effective for adult participants. In particular, those completing the program as graduates were less likely to immediately reoffend than nongraduates. Participants noted appreciation for the empathy element among program counselors and mentors and for the program's integration of cultural ties and justice principles. Beyond the participants, their families and community at large deemed the program to be successful.

As the data and trends discussed in this chapter illustrate, a multisectoral approach is needed to comprehensively address public health needs of Indigenous people who are impacted by incarceration. A multisectoral approach consists of institutions from several different sectors, including academia, nonprofits, public health, and local governments (especially tribal governments), collaborating toward a holistic view of local health outcomes. We believe that a multisectoral or collective impact framework is necessary to reduce the "broken" public health system in jails and prisons, which partially contributes to the health disparities affecting incarcerated Indigenous people. "Collective impact initiatives are long-term commitments by a group of important actors from different sectors to a common agenda for solving a specific social problem with their actions supported by a shared measurement system, mutually reinforcing activities, and ongoing communication" (Camplain and Baldwin 2019, 47). While the aforementioned disparities between racial populations are known, the ability to develop mechanisms and pathways to address social determinants at critical intercepts, prior to criminal justice interaction, has continued to challenge policymakers. Thus, if scalable and sustainable progress is to be made, partnerships must be forged among separated and often siloed organizations and perspectives. An emerging population health framework that integrates a broad historical lens to identify systemic patterns of oppression at the community level and recognizes the role of the community ecosystem and its impacts on justice and health is fundamental.

REFERENCES

Australian Bureau of Statistics. 2022. "Australia: Aboriginal and Torres Strait Islander Population Summary." https://www.abs.gov.au/articles/australia-aboriginal-and-torres-strait-islander-population-summary.

Australian Bureau of Statistics. 2023. "Prisoners in Australia." https://www.abs.gov.au/statistics/people/crime-and-justice/prisoners-australia/latest-release.

Bai, Jennifer R., Montina Befus, Dhritiman V. Mukherjee, Franklin D. Lowy, and Elaine L. Larson. 2015. "Prevalence and Predictors of Chronic Health Conditions of Inmates Newly Admitted to Maximum Security Prisons." *Journal of Correctional Health Care* 21, no. 3: 255–64. https://doi.org/10.1177%2F1078345815587510.

Barger, Steven D., Matthew R. Cribbet, and Matthew F. Muldoon. 2016. "Participant-Reported Health Status Predicts Cardiovascular and All-Cause Mortality Independent of Established and Nontraditional Biomarkers: Evidence from a Representative US Sample." *Journal of the American Heart Association* 5, no. 9: e003741. https://doi.org/10.1161/JAHA.116.003741.

Barnes, J. C., Cody Jorgensen, Kevin M. Beaver, Brian B. Boutwell, and John P. Wright. 2015. "Arrest Prevalence in a National Sample of Adults: The Role of Sex and Race/Ethnicity." *American Journal of Criminal Justice* 40, no. 3: 457–65. https://doi.org/10.1007/s12103-014-9273-3.

Bazelon, Emily. 2020. *Charged: The New Movement to Transform American Prosecution and End Mass Incarceration*. New York: Random House.

Beals, Janette, Douglas K. Novins, Nancy R. Whitesell, Paul Spicer, Christina M. Mitchell, Spero M. Manson, and American Indian Service Utilization, Psychiatric Epidemiology, Risk and Protective Factors Project Team. 2005. "Prevalence of Mental Disorders and Utilization of Mental Health Services in Two

American Indian Reservation Populations: Mental Health Disparities in a National Context." *American Journal of Psychiatry* 162, no. 9: 1723–32. https://doi.org/10.1176/appi.ajp.162.9.1723.

BIA (Bureau of Indian Affairs). n.d. "Tribal Court Systems." Accessed March 11, 2023. https://www.bia.gov/CFRCourts/tribal-justice-support-directorate.

Binswanger, Ingrid A., Patrick M. Krueger, and John F. Steiner. 2009. "Prevalence of Chronic Medical Conditions Among Jail and Prison Inmates in the USA Compared with the General Population." *Journal of Epidemiology and Community Health* 63, no. 11: 912–19. https://doi.org/10.1136/jech.2009.090662.

Binswanger, Ingird A., N. Redmond, John F. Steiner, and LeRoi S. Hicks. 2012. "Health Disparities and the Criminal Justice System: An Agenda for Further Research and Action." *Journal of Urban Health* 89, no. 1: 98–107. https://doi.org/10.1007/s11524-011-9614-1.

BJA (Bureau of Justice Assistance). n.d. "Tribal Healing to Wellness Courts: Wellness Court Resources." Accessed June 7, 2022. http://wellnesscourts.org/wellness-court-resources/.

BJS (Bureau of Justice Statistics). n.d. "Jails in Indian Country." Bureau of Justice Statistics. Accessed March 9, 2023. https://bjs.ojp.gov/topics/tribal-crime-and-justice/jails-in-indian-country.

BJS (Bureau of Justice Statistics). 2018. "Terms and Definitions: Local Jail Inmates and Jail Facilities." https://www.bjs.gov/index.cfm?ty=tdtp&tid=12.

BJS (Bureau of Justice Statistics). 2021. "The Justice System." https://www.bjs.gov/content/justsys.cfm#contents.

Blankenship, Kim M., Ana Maria del Rio Gonzalez, Danya E. Keene, Allison K. Groves, and Alana P. Rosenberg. 2018. "Mass Incarceration, Race Inequality, and Health: Expanding Concepts and Assessing Impacts on Well-Being." *Social Science and Medicine* 215 (October): 45–52. https://doi.org/10.1016/j.socscimed.2018.08.042.

Bonczar, Thomas P. 2003. *Prevalence of Imprisonment in the US Population, 1974–2001*. Bureau of Justice Statistics Special Report, NCJ 197976. Washington, D.C.: Office of Justice Programs, August 2003. https://bjs.ojp.gov/content/pub/pdf/piusp01.pdf.

Braithwaite, John. 1999. "Restorative Justice: Assessing Optimistic and Pessimistic Accounts." *Crime and Justice* 25: 1–127. https://www.jstor.org/stable/1147608.

Brewer, Graham Lee. 2016. "In Oklahoma's Prison System, Native American Inmates Carry On Tradition." *Oklahoman*, December 25, 2016. https://www.oklahoman.com/article/5531943/in-oklahomas-prison-system-native-american-inmates-carry-on-tradition.

Bronson, Jennifer, and E. Ann Carson. 2019. *Prisoners in 2017.* Bureau of Justice Statistics Special Report, NCJ 252156. Washington, D.C.: Office of Justice Programs, April 2019. https://bjs.ojp.gov/content/pub/pdf/p17.pdf.

Brown, Jennifer. 2014. *Flagstaff Police Department Annual Report 2014.* Flagstaff, AZ: Flagstaff Police Department. https://prism.lib.asu.edu/_flysystem/fedora /c16/146208/2014_AnnualReport.pdf.

Brown, Toyacoyah. 2014. "Pow Wow Allows Inmates to Reconnect with Their Roots." PowWows.com. https://www.powwows.com/pow-wow-allows-in mates-to-reconnect-with-their-roots/.

Camplain, Ricky, and Julie A. Baldwin. 2019. "Commentary: The Search for Health Equity Among Individuals Incarcerated in Jail." *Practicing Anthropology* 41, no. 4: 46–48. https://doi.org/10.17730%2F0888-4552.41.4.46.

Camplain, Ricky, Julie A. Baldwin, Meghan Warren, Carolyn Camplain, Monica R. Lininger, and Robert T. Trotter. 2019. "Physical Activity in People Who Are Incarcerated: A Social Justice Issue." *Journal of Physical. Activity and Health* 16, no. 5: 306–7. https://doi.org/10.1123/jpah.2019-0055.

Camplain, Ricky, Lyle Becenti, Travis A. Pinn, Heather J. Williamson, George Pro, Crystal Luna, and James Bret. 2022. "Physical Activity Patterns Among Women Incarcerated in Jail." *Journal of Correctional Health Care* 28, no. 1: 6–11. https://doi.org/10.1089/jchc.20.05.0041.

Camplain, Ricky, Carolyn Camplain, Robert T. Trotter, George Pro, Samantha Sabo, Emery Eaves, Marie Peoples, and Julie A. Baldwin. 2020. "Racial/Ethnic Differences in Drug-and Alcohol-Related Arrest Outcomes in a Southwest County from 2009 to 2018." *American Journal of Public Health* 110, no. S1: S85–92. https://doi.org/10.2105/AJPH.2019.305409.

Camplain, Ricky, Meghan Warren, Julie A. Baldwin, Carolyn Camplain, Viacheslav Y. Fofanov, and Robert T. Trotter. 2019. "Epidemiology of Incarceration: Characterizing Jail Incarceration for Public Health Research." *Epidemiology* 30, no. 4: 561–68. https://doi.org/10.1097%2FEDE.0000000000001021.

Casey, Rachel C.. 2020. "Healing Circles in Maine Prisons: Connecting Native People with Community and Culture." Maine-Wabanaki REACH, February 5, 2020. https://www.wabanakireach.org/healing_circles_in_maine_prisons.

Chaddock, Don. 2018. "Native American Spiritual Leaders, Recruiters at Capitol." California Department of Corrections and Rehabilitation, October 3, 2018. https://www.cdcr.ca.gov/insidecdcr/2018/10/03/cdcr-native-american -spiritual-leaders/.

Conley, Timothy B., and David L. Schantz. 2006. *Predicting and Reducing Recidivism: Factors Contributing to Recidivism in the State of Montana Pre-Release Center Population and the Issue of Measurement: A Report with Recommendations for Policy Change.* Missoula: University of Montana, School of Social Work. https://leg.mt.gov/content/committees/interim/2007_2008/law_justice/meeting_documents/DOC%20report%2011-21-06.pdf.

CSG (Council of State Governments) Justice Center. 2015. *Justice Reinvestment in Montana: Overview.* New York: Council of State Governments Justice Center, November 2015. https://csgjusticecenter.org/publications/justice-reinvestment-in-montana-overview/.

Cunningham, James K., Teshia A. Solomon, and Myra L. Muramoto. 2016. "Alcohol Use Among Native Americans Compared to Whites: Examining the Veracity of the 'Native American Elevated Alcohol Consumption' Belief." *Drug and Alcohol Dependence* 160 (March): 65–75. https://doi.org/10.1016/j.drugalcdep.2015.12.015.

Daniel, Roxanne. 2020. "Since You Asked: What Data Exists about Native American People in the Criminal Justice System?" Prison Policy Initiative, April 22, 2020. https://www.prisonpolicy.org/blog/2020/04/22/native/.

Department of Justice Canada. 2023. "Overrepresentation of Indigenous People in the Canadian Criminal Justice System: Causes and Responses." https://www.justice.gc.ca/eng/rp-pr/jr/oip-cjs/p3.html.

Echo-Hawk, Walter. 1996. *Study of Native American Prisoner Issues.* Washington, D.C.: National Indian Policy Center, George Washington University.

Fazel, Seena, and John Danesh. 2002. "Serious Mental Disorder in 23000 Prisoners: A Systematic Review of 62 Surveys." *Lancet* 359 (9306): 545–50. https://doi.org/10.1016/s0140-6736(02)07740-1.

Feldstein, Sarah W., and Joel I. D. Ginsburg. 2006. "Motivational Interviewing with Dually Diagnosed Adolescents in Juvenile Justice Settings." *Brief Treatment and Crisis Intervention* 6, no. 3: 218–33. https://psycnet.apa.org/doi/10.1093/brief-treatment/mhl003.

Feldstein, Sarah W., Kamilla L. Venner, and Philip A. May. 2006. "American Indian/Alaska Native Alcohol-Related Incarceration and Treatment." *American Indian and Alaska Native Mental Health Research (Online)* 13, no. 3: 1–22. https://doi.org/10.5820%2Faian.1303.2006.1.

Flies-Away, Joseph Thomas, Jerry Gardner, and Carrie Garrow. 2014. *Overview of Tribal Healing to Wellness Courts.* 2nd ed. West Hollywood: Tribal Law and Policy Institute. http://www.wellnesscourts.org/files/THWC%20Overview%20Final%20-%20Sept%20%202014.pdf.

Flies-Away, Joseph Thomas, Carrie Garrow, and Pat Sekaquaptewa. 2014. *Tribal Healing to Wellness Courts: The Key Components.* 2nd ed. West Hollywood: Tribal Law and Policy Institute, September 2014. http://www.wellnesscourts.org/files/Tribal%20Healing%20to%20Wellness%20Courts%20The%20Key%20Components.pdf.

Garrett, Michael T'lanusta, Edil Torres-Rivera, Michael Brubaker, Tarrell Awe Agahe Portman, Dale Brotherton, Cirecie West-Olatunji, William Conwill, and Lisa Grayshield. 2011. "Crying for a Vision: The Native American Sweat Lodge Ceremony as Therapeutic Intervention." *Journal of Counseling and Development* 89, no. 3: 318–25. https://doi.org/10.1002/j.1556-6678.2011.tb00096.x.

George, Blythe. 2020. "Prisoner Re-Entry in Native American Communities Offers Lessons of Resilience and Nationwide Policy Solutions." Washington Center for Equitable Growth, February 18, 2020. https://equitablegrowth.org /prisoner-re-entry-in-native-american-communities-offers-lessons-of-resili ence-and-nationwide-policy-solutions/.

Gone, Joseph P., and Joseph E. Trimble. 2012. "American Indian and Alaska Native Mental Health: Diverse Perspectives on Enduring Disparities." *Annual Review of Clinical Psychology* 8: 131–60. https://doi.org/10.1146/annurev-clin psy-032511-143127.

Gonzalez, Vivian M., and Monica C. Skewes. 2016. "Association of the Firewater Myth with Drinking Behavior Among American Indian and Alaska Native College Students." *Psychology of Addictive Behaviors* 30, no. 8: 838–49. https:// doi.org/10.1037/adb0000226.

Gorsuch, Marina M., and Deborah T. Rho. 2019. "Police Stops and Searches of Indigenous People in Minneapolis: The Roles of Race, Place, and Gender." *International Indigenous Policy Journal* 10, no. 3: 1–28. https://doi.org/10.18584 /iipj.2019.10.3.8322.

Gossage, J. Phillip, Louie Barton, Lenny Foster, Larry Etsitty, Clayton LoneTree, Carol Leonard, and Philip A. May. 2003. "Sweat Lodge Ceremonies for Jail-Based Treatment." *Journal of Psychoactive Drugs* 35, no. 1: 33–42. https://doi .org/10.1080/02791072.2003.10399991.

Gottlieb, Karen. 2005. *Process and Outcome Evaluations in Four Tribal Wellness Courts.* NCJ 231167. Washington, D.C.: Office of Justice Programs, December 2005. https://www.ojp.gov/library/publications/process-and-outcome-evalu ations-four-tribal-wellness-courts.

Greenfeld, Lawrence A., and Steven K. Smith. 1999. *American Indians and Crime.* Bureau of Justice Statistics report, NCJ 173386. Washington, D.C.: Office of Justice Programs, February 1999. https://bjs.ojp.gov/content/pub/pdf/aic.pdf.

Hartney, Christopher, and Linh Vuong. 2009. *Created Equal: Racial and Ethnic Disparities in the US Criminal Justice System.* Oakland: National Council on Crime and Delinquency. http://www.racialviolenceus.org/Articles/created-equal.pdf.

Haywood, Phaedra. 2019. "Honoring Native Traditions Behind Bars." *Santa Fe New Mexican*, December 28, 2019. https://www.santafenewmexican.com/news /local_news/honoring-native-traditions-behind-bars/article_47a591d0-1aeb -11ea-b592-c7dd4f4b25ad.html.

HHS (U.S. Department of Health and Human Services). 2001. *Mental Health: Culture, Race, and Ethnicity—A Supplement to Mental Health: A Report of The Surgeon General*. Washington, D.C.: U.S. Public Health Service, August 2001. https://www.ncbi.nlm.nih.gov/books/NBK44243/.

Hopper, Frank. 2021. "The Pandemic in Prison: How COVID Robbed Native Inmates of Vital Cultural and Spiritual Support." Last Real Indians, March 2, 2021. https://lastrealindians.com/news/2021/3/2/the-pandemic-in-prison-how-covid-robbed-native-inmates-of-vital-cultural-and-spiritual-support-by-frank-hopper.

Hutchinson, Rebecca Newlin, and Sonya Shin. 2014. "Systematic Review of Health Disparities for Cardiovascular Diseases and Associated Factors Among American Indian and Alaska Native Populations." *PloS ONE* 9, no. 1: e80973. https://doi.org/10.1371/journal.pone.0080973.

Irwin, Lee. 2006. "Walking the Line: Pipe and Sweat Ceremonies in Prison." *Nova Religio* 9, no. 3: 39–60. https://doi.org/10.1525/nr.2006.9.3.039.

Jones, Alexi. 2018. "Correctional Control 2018: Incarceration and Supervision by State." Prison Policy Initiative, December 2018. https://www.prisonpolicy.org/reports/correctionalcontrol2018.html.

Jones, David S. 2006. "The Persistence of American Indian Health Disparities." *American Journal of Public Health* 96, no. 12 (December): 2122–34. https://doi.org/10.2105%2FAJPH.2004.054262.

Kochel, Tammy Rinehart, David B. Wilson, and Stephen D. Mastrofski. 2011. "Effect of Suspect Race on Officers' Arrest Decisions." *Criminology* 49, no. 2: 473–512. https://doi.org/10.1111/j.1745-9125.2011.00230.x.

Lester, David. 1999. *Crime and the Native American*: Springfield, IL: Charles C. Thomas Publisher.

Maruschak, Laura M., Marcus Berzofsky, and Jennifer Unangst. 2015. *Medical Problems of State and Federal Prisoners and Jail Inmates, 2011–12*. Bureau of Justice Statistics Special Report, NCJ 248491. Washington, D.C.: U.S. Department of Justice, February 2015. https://bjs.ojp.gov/content/pub/pdf/mpsfpji1112.pdf.

Massoglia, Michael. 2008. "Incarceration as Exposure: The Prison, Infectious Disease, and Other Stress-Related Illnesses." *Journal Of Health and Social Behavior* 49, no. 1 (March): 56–71. https://doi.org/10.1177/002214650804900105.

Mauer, Marc, and Ryan S. King. 2007. *Uneven Justice: State Rates of Incarceration by Race and Ethnicity*. Washington, D.C.: Sentencing Project, January 2007. https://www.researchgate.net/publication/242491046_Uneven_Justice_State_Rates_of_Incarceration_By_Race_and_Ethnicity.

Metoui, Jessica. 2007. "Returning to the Circle: The Reemergence of Traditional Dispute Resolution in Native American Communities." *Journal of Dispute*

Resolution 2007, no. 2: 517–39. https://scholarship.law.missouri.edu/jdr/vol 2007/iss2/6.

Minton, Todd D., and Mary P. Cowhig. 2020. *Jails in Indian Country, 2017–2018*. Bureau of Justice Statistics report, NCJ 252155. Washington, D.C.: Office of Justice Programs, October 2020. https://bjs.ojp.gov/library/publications/jails -indian-country-2017-2018#:~:text=A%20total%20of%2084%20jails,from%2 04%2C200%20at%20midyear%202017.

Moore, Kelly. 2010. "Youth-Onset Type 2 Diabetes Among American Indians and Alaska Natives." *Journal of Public Health Management and Practice* 16, no. 5: 388–93. https://doi.org/10.1097/phh.0b013e3181cbc4b5.

Morgan, Oscar, Ford Kuramoto, William Emmet, Judy L. Stange, and Eeric Nobunaga. 2014. "The Impact of the Affordable Care Act on Behavioral Health Care for Individuals from Racial and Ethnic Communities." *Journal of Social Work in Disability and Rehabilitation* 13, no. 1–2: 139–61. https://doi.org/10 .1080/1536710X.2013.870518.

Mulia, Nina, Yu Ye, Sarah E. Zemore, and Thomas K. Greenfield. 2008. "Social Disadvantage, Stress, and Alcohol Use Among Black, Hispanic, and White Americans: Findings from the 2005 US National Alcohol Survey." *Journal of Studies on Alcohol and Drugs* 69, no. 6: 824–33. https://doi.org/10.15288 %2Fjsad.2008.69.824.

Native American Rights Fund. 2016. "Legal Protections for Native Spiritual Practices in Prison." https://narf.org/nill/documents/2016_protections_pri soners.pdf.

NCAI (National Congress of American Indians). n.d. "Tribal Law & Order Act." Accessed March 11, 2023. https://www.ncai.org/tribal-vawa/resources/tribal -law-order-act.

Nielsen, Marianne O., and Linda M. Robyn. 2019. *Colonialism Is Crime*. New Brunswick, NJ: Rutgers University Press.

Niveau, G. 2006. "Prevention of Infectious Disease Transmission in Correctional Settings: A Review." *Public Health* 120, no. 1 (January): 33–41. https://doi.org /10.1016/j.puhe.2005.03.017.

Parks, Bradley W., and Arya Surowidjojo. 2020. "Indigenous Inmates, Volunteers Navigate a Year Without Ceremonies, Celebrations." Oregon Public Broad-casting, December 14, 2020. https://www.opb.org/article/2020/12/14/native -american-religious-services-oregon-prison-covid-19/.

Perry, Steven W. 2004. *American Indians and Crime: A BJS Statistical Profile, 1992– 2002*. Bureau of Justice Statistics, NCJ 203097. Washington, D.C.: Office of Justice Programs, December 2004. https://bjs.ojp.gov/library/publications /american-indians-and-crime-bjs-statistical-profile-1992-2002.

Puglisi, Lisa, Joseph P. Calderon, and Emily A. Wang. 2017. "What Does Health Justice Look Like for People Returning from Incarceration?" *AMA Journal of Ethics* 19, no. 9: 903–10. http://dx.doi.org/10.1001/journalofethics.2017.19.9 .ecas4-1709.

Red Road. 2021. "Substance Abuse and Native Americans." https://theredroad .org/issues/native-american-substance-abuse/.

Reha, Bob. 2001. "Spiritual Freedom Behind Bars." Minnesota Public Radio, April 2001. http://news.minnesota.publicradio.org/projects/2001/04/broken trust/rehab_spiritual-m/index.shtml.

Ross, Luana. 1998. *Inventing the Savage: The Social Construction of Native American Criminality.* Austin: University of Texas Press.

Sakala, Leah. 2014. "Breaking Down Mass Incarceration in the 2010 Census: State-By-State Incarceration Rates by Race/Ethnicity." Prison Policy Initiative, May 28, 2014. https://www.prisonpolicy.org/reports/rates.html.

Sawyer, Wendy, and Peter Wagner. 2020. "Mass Incarceration: The Whole Pie 2020." Prison Policy Initiative, March 24, 2020. https://www.prisonpolicy.org /factsheets/pie2020_allimages.pdf.

Snyder, Howard N. 2011. *Arrest in the United States, 1980–2009.* Bureau of Justice Statistics report, NCJ 234319. Washington, D.C.: Office of Justice Programs, September 2011. https://bjs.ojp.gov/content/pub/pdf/aus8009.pdf.

Spicer, Paul, Janette Beals, Calvin D. Croy, Christina M. Mitchell, Douglas K. Novins, Laurie Moore, and Spero M. Manson. 2003. "The Prevalence of DSM-III-R Alcohol Dependence in Two American Indian Populations." *Alcoholism: Clinical and Experimental Research* 27, no. 11 (November): 1785–97. https://doi .org/10.1097/01.alc.0000095864.45755.53.

Statista. 2022. "Number of Arrests for All Offenses in the United States from 1990 to 2019." Statista Research Department, October 2022. https://www .statista.com/statistics/191261/number-of-arrests-for-all-offenses-in-the-us -since-1990/.

Steele, Paul, Nell Damon, and Kristine Denman. 2004. *Crime and the New Mexico Reservation: An Analysis of Crime on Native American Land (1996–2002), Final Report.* Albuquerque: New Mexico Criminal Justice Analysis Center, University of New Mexico Institute for Social Research, October 2004. https://www .ojp.gov/pdffiles1/bjs/grants/212238.pdf.

Tighe, Scott. 2014. "'Of Course We Are Crazy': Discrimination of Native American Indians Through Criminal Justice." *Justice Policy Journal* 11, no. 1 (Spring): 1–38. https://www.cjcj.org/media/import/documents/tighe_discrimination _final_formatted.pdf.

Tribal Law and Policy Institute. 2003. *Tribal Healing to Wellness Courts: The Key Components*. Bureau of Justice Assistance report, NCJ 188154. Washington, D.C.: Office of Justice Programs, April 2003. https://www.ojp.gov/pdffiles1 /bja/188154.pdf.

Tribal Law and Policy Institute. 2017. *Healing to Wellness Courts: Treatment Guidelines*. 2nd ed. West Hollywood: Tribal Law and Policy Institute, November 2017. https://www.wicourts.gov/courts/programs/problemsolving/docs/treat mentguide.pdf.

Trotter, Robert T., Ricky Camplain, Emery R. Eaves, Viacheslav Y. Fofanov, Natalia O. Dmitrieva, Crystal M. Hepp, Meghan Warren, Brianna A. Barrios, Nicole Pagel, Alyssa Mayer, and Julie A. Baldwin. 2018. "Health Disparities and Converging Epidemics in Jail Populations: Protocol for a Mixed-Methods Study." *JMIR Research Protocols* 7, no. 10 (October): e10337. https://doi.org/10 .2196/10337.

Trotter, Robert T., Monica R. Lininger, Ricky Camplain, Viacheslav Y. Fofanov, Carolyn Camplain, and Julie A. Baldwin. 2018. "A Survey of Health Disparities, Social Determinants of Health, and Converging Morbidities in a County Jail: A Cultural-Ecological Assessment of Health Conditions in Jail Populations." *International Journal of Environmental Research and Public Health* 15, no. 11: 2500. https://doi.org/10.3390/ijerph15112500.

U.S. Sentencing Commission. 2013. "Native Americans in the Federal Offender Population." Quick Facts. https://www.ussc.gov/sites/default/files /pdf/research-and-publications/quick-facts/Quick_Facts_Native_American _Offenders.pdf.

Waldram, J. B. 2020. "Aboriginal Spirituality in Corrections." In *Native Americans, Crime, and Justice*, edited by Marianne O. Nielsen and Robert A. Silverman, 239–53. Abingdon, UK: Routledge.

Walmsley, Roy. 2018. *World Prison Population List, Twelfth Edition*. London, UK: Institute for Criminal Policy Research.

Washington State Department of Corrections. 2020. "Tribal Relations." https:// www.doc.wa.gov/about/agency/tribal.htm.

Wellbriety Circles. 2021. "White Bison." https://whitebison.org/WellBriety.aspx.

Wiggins, Charles L., David K. Espey, Phyllis A. Wingo, Judith S. Kaur, Robin Taylor Wilson, Judith Swan, Barry A. Miller, Melissa A. Jim, Janet J. Kelly, and Anne P. Lanier. 2008. "Cancer Among American Indians and Alaska Natives in The United States, 1999–2004." *Cancer: Interdisciplinary International Journal of the American Cancer Society* 113, no. S1 (September): 1142–52. https:// doi.org/10.1002/cncr.23734.

Wilper, Andrew P., Steffie Woolhandler, J. Wesley Boyd, Karen E. Lasser, Danny McCormick, David H. Bor, and David U. Himmelstein. 2009. "The Health and Health Care of US Prisoners: Results of a Nationwide Survey." *American Journal Of Public Health* 99, no. 4 (April): 666–72. https://doi.org/10.2105%2F AJPH.2008.144279.

Winick, Bruce J. 2013. "Problem Solving Courts: Therapeutic Jurisprudence in Practice." In *Problem Solving Courts: Social Science and Legal Perspectives*, edited by R. L. Wiener and E. M. Brank, 211–36. New York: Springer.

Wu, Jawjeong. 2016. "Racial/Ethnic Discrimination and Prosecution: A Meta-Analysis." *Criminal Justice and Behavior* 43, no. 4: 437–58. https://psycnet.apa .org/doi/10.1177/0093854815628026.

Yang, Hong, and Julian R. Thompson. 2020. "Fighting COVID-19 Outbreaks in Prisons." *BMJ* 369, no. 1362. https://doi.org/10.1136/bmj.m1362.

Zehr, Howard. 1990. *Changing Lenses: A New Focus for Crime and Justice*. Scottdale, PA: Herald Press.

Zeng, Zhen. 2018. *Jail Inmates in 2016*. Bureau of Justice Statistics bulletin, NCJ 251210. Washington, D.C.: Office of Justice Programs, February 2018. https:// bjs.ojp.gov/content/pub/pdf/ji16.pdf.

LEGAL RESOURCES

American Indian Religious Freedom, Pub. L. No. 95–341, 92 Stat. 469 (1978)

Indian Citizenship Act, Pub. L. No. 68–175, 43 Stat. 253 (1924)

Religious Freedom Restoration Act, Pub. L. No. 103–141, 107 Stat. 1488 (1993)

Religious Land Use and Institutionalized Persons Act, Pub. L. No. 106–274, 114 Stat. 803 (2000)

Tribal Law and Order Act, Pub. L. No. 111–211, 124 Stat. 2258 (2010)

Wolff v. McDonnell, 418 U.S. 539 (1974)

2

THE HISTORICAL FAILURE OF THE INDIAN HEALTH SERVICE AND THE RESTORATION OF HEALTH-CARE SOVEREIGNTY

JOSEPH DIETRICH AND JEAN REITH SCHROEDEL

I N THIS CHAPTER, we[1] trace federally provided Native American health care from its inception in the early 1800s to the current era, considering its evolution, successes, and failures. The arrival of Europeans brought many new diseases, most notably measles and smallpox, that devastated Native populations. Since traditional medicines and practices were unable to treat white man's diseases, tribes sought to gain access to Western medicine, not to supplant traditional health practices but to use in conjunction with them. However, this was not the approach undertaken by the federal government, which as we show has a trust responsibility to provide health care to American Indian and Alaska Native populations. Instead, in 1955, the United States saddled tribes with an inefficient, poorly funded, and poorly managed health-care bureaucracy, which stifled tribal input regarding administration, to replace a series of other poorly run, inefficient bureaucracies that oversaw the provision of health care to tribes in the United States. In the following pages, we show how the federal government's role in the provision of health care has changed over time and in response to Native activism, which has pushed to establish a system that respects tribal authority and traditional healing practices. This has been an evolutionary process, which is far from complete. We do not ignore the

---

1. The authors wish to thank Kara Mazareas for her contributions to the development of this chapter.

shortcomings of the Indian Health Service (IHS) in this chapter, as we provide a detailed and expansive history of government-provided tribal health care, including abuses such as those occurring at the Quentin N. Burdick Memorial Health Care Facility on the Turtle Mountain Reservation and Sioux San Hospital in Rapid City. However, we end with a reflection on the status of self-determination today, noting that some tribes have used changes in federal law and policy to improve health care via mechanisms of local control.

At its establishment in 1955, the IHS was charged to 1) assemble a competent health staff, 2) institute extensive curative treatment for the seriously ill, and 3) develop a full-scale prevention program that would reduce the excessive amount of illness and early deaths among Native populations, especially for preventable diseases (IHS 1985). Over a half century later, none of these initial priorities has been fully achieved. IHS facilities are routinely understaffed and have a shortage of board-qualified specialists (GAO 2018). Curative treatments at IHS facilities are often unavailable or far inferior to treatment at local non-IHS facilities. Based on numbers from fiscal years 2017 and 2019, congressional appropriations met only 42 percent of Native American and Alaska Native health-care needs ($4,078 per person) when compared to health-care expenditures in the general U.S. population ($9,726 per person)—which is significantly healthier (IHS 2020).

This lack of quality care and adequate funding has contributed to and exacerbated disparate health outcomes over time. Diabetes, suicide, alcoholism and drug abuse, domestic violence and victimization, and heart disease have all risen or remained high among Native populations since 1980. American Indians have a 37 percent higher chance of dying from pneumonia and flu than the average U.S. population. More than 50 out of every 100,000 Native Americans will die of alcohol-related illness, whereas only 8 per 100,000 of all Americans will suffer the same fate (IHS 2015). Native women experience the highest rate of domestic violence (46 percent) and over one in three have been raped in their lifetime (37 percent) (Breiding, Chen, and Black 2014; Tjaden and Thoennes 1998). Native Americans have a lower life expectancy—more than five years shorter—than all other racial and ethnic groups (Adakai et al. 2018, 1314–18). COVID-19 hit Indian Country particularly hard. This underscores the importance of access to quality health-care services. Beyond these failures to meet its stated goals is a long list of abuses, malpractice, inferior facilities, and cover-ups at the IHS that stem from these underlying factors.

A HISTORY OF INDIAN HEALTH AND
THE FEDERAL GOVERNMENT

The federal government's responsibility for providing health care to Native populations is legally based on commitments made in treaties between the U.S. government and Native nations (see DeJong 2015) and reaffirmed in Supreme Court rulings and federal statutes. Although some early treaties were friendship pacts, the vast majority of treaties were aimed at opening land for non-Native settlement. In exchange for giving up tribal lands, the federal government made commitments to provide services—typically housing, education, and economic development—to tribal members and to protect their lands and resources (USCCR 2018). From 1836 onward, treaties typically included language committing the U.S. government to provide medical supplies and physicians to tribes (Shelton 2004).

The act of entering into treaties carries with it an implicit recognition that each party is a distinct and sovereign entity (Schroedel 2020, 14–15). The United States Constitution, in article 1, section 8, explicitly acknowledges the distinct sovereignty of Native nations in its description of Congress's power to regulate commerce with "foreign Nations, and among the several States, and with the Indian Tribes" (see Rife and Dellapenna 2009). This understanding that the federal government has a government-to-government relationship with Native nations has been further developed in Supreme Court decisions, most notably the Marshall Trilogy—*Johnson v. M'Intosh* (1823), *Cherokee Nation v. Georgia* (1831), and *Worcester v. Georgia* (1832). These court cases develop the federal trust doctrine, which affirmed that the federal government had control over Indian affairs and tribes were not bound by state regulations. Furthermore, in *Cherokee Nation v. Georgia*, Chief Justice John Marshall described tribes as "domestic dependent nations," with the federal-tribal relationship being akin to "that of a ward to his guardian." This ruling meant that the federal government could take lands from the tribes but that the federal government would be obligated to protect the tribes in the new lands and provide necessities such as food, housing, medical care, and education—all aimed in the first half of the nineteenth century at assimilating Native peoples into white ways of living.

Responsibility for Indian affairs was under the jurisdiction of the U.S. Department of War's Office of Indian Affairs. One of the first instances of the federal government taking direct responsibility for Native health occurred in 1832 with the passage of the Indian Vaccination Act, which tasked the military with vaccinating tribes in the southeastern states against smallpox. This was part of the federal government's efforts, under President Andrew Jackson, to forcibly relocate the Cherokee, Muscogee, Seminole, Chickasaw, and Choctaw to west of the Mississippi River to Indian Territory (now Oklahoma). The 1828 discovery of gold in northern Georgia increased white settlement in the region, which resulted in increased conflicts with the Indigenous inhabitants (Cherokee Nation 2023). Secretary of War Lewis Cass was given full authority over the program with no input from American Indians during the conception, design, or implementation (Pearson 2003). This effort continued during the first half of the nineteenth century, but the focus on preventing the spread of infectious diseases was aimed at protecting military outposts and settlers living near tribal lands (Shelton 2004).

In 1849, the Office of Indian Affairs was moved to the newly created U.S. Department of the Interior and, through "An Act to Establish the Home Department," the name was changed to the Bureau of Indian Affairs (BIA). Although the BIA oversaw the building of some health facilities on Indian reservations, they lacked the resources needed to combat infectious diseases, such as tuberculosis, trachoma, and smallpox, which were serious problems (NLM 2012). Moreover, a significant part of the U.S. government's efforts in the latter part of the nineteenth century was directed at militarily defeating Native nations who were fighting to keep their lands in the plains and Southwest from settler incursions. They were not interested in providing health services to peoples who they might subsequently be fighting. For example, in 1880, there were only seventy-seven doctors providing medical and health care through the BIA (Shelton 2004). They also were paid much lower salaries (less than 40 percent) of what military physicians were paid (Warne and Frizzell 2014).

By the beginning of the twentieth century, the health of Native populations had declined precipitously. The forced movement of tribes onto reservations separated people from their traditional sources of food and medicine, leaving them dependent on government-provided food staples that undermined their physical health. This combined with the banning of traditional medicine and healing ceremonies, again all part of the federal government's assimilation policy, had deleterious effects on people's well-being (Shelton 2004; Kuschell-Haworth 2010).

ESTABLISHING AN INDIAN HEALTH SERVICE

Prior to 1921, the BIA did not have an ongoing budget for the provision of health services to Native Americans. Instead, each project had to be separately approved and funded by congressional legislation. This changed with the 1921 passage of the Snyder Act, which authorized general expenditures for "the relief of distress and conservation of health" among American Indians. The legislation also linked the BIA's activities to congressional appropriations by providing for the use of "such monies as Congress may from time to time appropriate, for the benefit, care, and assistance of Indians" (Rhoades, Reyes, and Buzzard 1987). While an important step forward, the act did not guarantee access to specific medical services (Rhoades, Reyes, and Buzzard 1987). These shortcomings received substantial attention in the 1928 report *The Problem of Indian Administration* (known as the Meriam Report), which found the following: "The health of the Indians as compared with the general population is bad. Although accurate mortality and morbidity statistics are commonly lacking, the existing evidence warrants the statement that both the general death rate and the infant mortality rate are high. Tuberculosis is extremely prevalent. Trachoma, a communicable disease which produces blindness, is a major problem because of its great prevalence and the danger of its spreading among both the Indians and the whites" (Meriam 1928).

In 1933, a reformer named John Collier was appointed to head the BIA. The following year, he convinced Congress to pass two important acts that resulted in significant changes for tribal governments seeking a greater role in decisions impacting their tribes. The first of these, the Johnson-O'Malley Act of 1934, allowed the BIA to contract out health services with states and territories. This provided a means for overcoming some of the shortages in medical services. The second one, the Indian

Reorganization Act of 1934, allowed tribal governments to have some degree of control over economic development and regain some of the lands that had been expropriated in prior decades. Unfortunately, federal government policies shifted against self-determination starting in the late 1940s with laws designed to promote rapid assimilation through the termination of federal recognition, forced sale of tribal lands, and the denial of treaty-promised services, including health care (Schroedel 2020, 27; Wilkins and Stark 2011, 130–31). Congress also passed laws aimed at moving Native people away from rural areas, including tribal lands, and relocating them into urban centers. Meanwhile, according to a 1949 American Medical Association report, tuberculosis rates on the Navajo Nation were ten times higher than among the general population (Moorman 1949).

Frustrated by the BIA's continuing failure to effectively address Indian health disparities, an administrative reshuffling occurred. Congress transferred the provision of health care to the Commissioned Corps of the Public Health Service (USPHS), which was part of the U.S. Department of Health, Education, and Welfare (HEW). HEW evolved into the current U.S. Department of Health and Human Services (HHS) in 1979 upon the creation of the separate U.S. Department of Education. Under HEW, the Division of Indian Health (renamed the Indian Health Service in 1958) took over the provision of direct medical and public health services to members of federally recognized tribes and Alaska Natives. In 1957, the USPHS submitted a report to Congress (St.J. Perrott and West 1957). This report found that among American Indians, total mortality was 20 percent higher, infant mortality was three times higher, life expectancy was ten years lower, and infectious diseases were more prevalent than what would be found in the general population (Jones 2006; St. J. Perrott and West 1957).

The appropriation was doubled and the IHS began training staff in "cross-cultural medicine" (Rhoades and Rhoades 2014). Congress also provided funding and authorization for the IHS to construct sanitation facilities on tribal lands (Public Law 86–121, 1959). The law required the participation of reservation communities to make decisions about the building and operation of the facilities, which established a precedent for the joint management of health programs. These shifts toward a more respectful stance vis-à-vis tribal governments and respect for traditional healing was an outgrowth of the success of the Many Farms Demonstration Project, a collaborative effort including the Navajo Nation, the USPHS, the IHS, and Cornell University Medical College that integrated traditional healing practices along with allopathic medicine (Rhoades 2009).

The result of these changes was marked improvements in the health of Native Americans (Lawrence 2000). Slowly, the sanitation issues that had plagued reservation lands for decades began to be addressed with modern facilities. General health care improved. During the first twenty-five years after control was given over to the USPHS, there were dramatic drops in the rates of infant mortality (82 percent), maternal deaths (89 percent), and tuberculosis mortality (96 percent) (Rhoades, D'Angelo, and Hurlburt 1987). However, so long as termination was the goal of federal government policy, all of these improvements were at risk of ending at any time.

THE STRUGGLE FOR SELF-DETERMINATION

World War II had an enormous impact on Native political activism. After fighting for the country, returning Native veterans, like Black veterans, felt their service had earned them full citizenship rights. Also, by bringing together men from different tribes, military service contributed to the creation of a common Native identity. Out of this newfound identity, the National Congress of American Indians (NCAI) was created to engage in lobbying government bureaucracies and Congress from 1944 onward (Smith and Warrior 1996).

During the termination era from 1953 through 1968, the policy was, as former U.S. senator Ben Nighthorse Campbell described, "If you can't change them, absorb them until they simply disappear into the mainstream culture. . . . In Washington's infinite wisdom, it was decided that tribes should no longer be tribes, never mind that they had been tribes for thousands of years" (Nighthorse Campbell 2007). As a result of the existential threat to their culture, Native Americans' resistance to federal government policies aimed at the expropriation of lands and the termination of treaty rights skyrocketed in the 1960s with increasing Native calls for self-determination and Red Power. One of the first calls for self-determination and Indigenous rights was the 1961 *Declaration of Indian*

Purpose (AICC 1961). The National Indian Youth Council, a national college youth organization, coined the phrase "Red Power," which subsequently was popularized by the American Indian Movement (AIM) and those involved in fish-ins designed to protect treaty rights to fishing (Blansett 2018; Reinhardt 2007; Smith and Warrior 1996).

Responding to this pressure, President Richard Nixon in 1970 endorsed the reversal of termination policies and called for a new policy of "self-determination without termination," instigating lasting changes in federal-Indian relationships, including the restoration of some tribal lands, programs for urban Indians, the creation of a cabinet-level position for Indian affairs, and the expansion of health-care programs (Landry 2016). However, the IHS continued to be underfunded and experienced staff shortages and high turnover. During the 1970s, life expectancy of Native Americans was one-third shorter than the national average; the incidence of poor outcomes such as infant mortality (1.5 times), diabetes (2 times), suicide (3 times), accidents (4 times), tuberculosis (14 times), gastrointestinal infections (27 times), dysentery (40 times), and rheumatic fever (60 times) was much greater than the national average (Jones 2006). There also were accusations that the IHS was performing involuntary sterilizations on Native women, which were subsequently verified by studies (Lawrence 2000).

HEALTH-CARE SOVEREIGNTY FOR TRIBES

The secretary of the HHS and the director of the IHS have the most direct control of policy within the IHS; reform therefore begins within their offices. However, Congress also has a duty to ensure that these institutions are serving their constituents. It could act on this issue by passing legislation directing IHS or the HHS to institute necessary and needed reforms. During the mid-1970s, they did so by passing a number of laws that enhanced the sovereignty of Native nations. Some laws only affected specific tribes, such as laws that returned sovereignty and federal recognition to some of tribes that had been terminated. Two laws, the 1975 Indian Self-Determination and Education Assistance Act (ISDEAA) and the 1976 Indian Health Care Improvement Act (IHCIA), had much broader effects on health-care sovereignty.

The ISDEAA states that the secretaries of the Interior and HHS can, at the request of tribal leaders, enter into contracts with tribal organizations to take over programs that had previously been under the control of federal government entities. This provided a mechanism for initially a limited number of tribes to manage health programs and receive a larger portion of IHS funding (Shelton 2004). The act, as well as the demonstration projects, were made subject to renewal, which occurred in 1994 when they were made permanent, and the number of projects expanded through the Tribal Self-Governance Act of 1994.

The initial 1976 IHCIA, which allowed the IHS to bill Medicare, Medicaid, and other insurers such as the State Children's Health Insurance Program and the U.S. Department of Veterans Affairs, brought new financial stability to Native American health services (CRS 2014). The IHCIA provided funding for programs providing services to urban Indians, the recruitment of health-care professionals, substance abuse treatment, and mental health services. It allowed for the creation of tribal-specific health plans (CRS 2014). The IHCIA provisions were made permanent in 2010 as part of the Affordable Care Act. In discussing these provisions, HHS secretary Kathleen Sebelius stated this was part of the federal government's commitment to "honoring the obligations of our government-to-government relationship with American Indian tribes, including the promise of adequate health care" (IHS 2010).

THE INDIAN HEALTH SERVICE TODAY

The IHS currently serves 2.56 million American Indians and Alaska Natives from 574 federally recognized tribes (IHS 2020), but the ways that it fulfills its trust responsibility is radically different than in the past. The current health-care delivery system is described as an "I/T/U system," where the letter "I" stands for IHS-delivered care, "T" stands for services delivered by tribes, and "U" stands for the thirty-four urban health programs (Warne and Frizzell 2014). There also is much more collaboration between tribal governments, the IHS, and other government entities, such as the Centers for Disease Control and Prevention and the National Institutes of Health, as well as with health organizations, such as the American Heart Association (Rhoades and Rhoades 2014).

While there have been improvements over time in the federal government's provision of health care to American Indian and Alaska Native populations, there are still serious shortcomings. An obvious and long-standing issue is the severe underfunding of service providers. Since IHS funding is discretionary rather than treated as an entitlement, it must be reappropriated annually and is subject to political pressures. In the 1990s, the per capita funding for IHS programs had a funding shortfall of 46 percent compared to the standard established for the Federal Employees Health Benefits Program (Warne and Frizzell 2014). In 2017, IHS per capita spending was $4,078, compared to $8,109 for Medicaid, $10,692 for health care at the U.S. Department of Veterans Affairs, and $13,185 for Medicare (Frieden 2020).

There also have been administrative difficulties. In 2009, Dr. Yvette Roubideaux, a member of the Rosebud Sioux Tribe, was appointed director of the IHS, but she was not confirmed by the Senate for a second term in 2013. Roubideaux had pushed for the permanent reauthorization of the IHCIA, but she spent much of her time in battles over getting tribal self-determination contract costs fully covered (Indianz.com 2015). After Roubideaux stepped down, the IHS entered into a period of extreme instability with a mix of directors, acting directors, and interim directors—five in total. This lack of stable leadership has made it hard for the IHS to continue making progress in providing high-quality health care to patients.

THE DORGAN REPORT

At no time was the endemic lack of funding and instability in leadership more obvious and directly felt than with the 2010 release of *In Critical Condition: The Urgent Need to Reform the Indian Health Service's Aberdeen Area*, which came to be known as the Dorgan Report (SCIA 2010b). The Aberdeen area, today referred to by the IHS as the Great Plains area, at the time included twenty facilities serving eighteen tribes in South Dakota, North Dakota, Nebraska, and Iowa. Then chairman of the Senate Committee on Indian Affairs, Senator Byron Dorgan (D-ND), released the report following an investigation that included a review of more than 140,000 pages of documents from the IHS and from the HHS's Office of Inspector General, visits to three local facilities, meetings with tribal members and facility employees throughout the region, and the input of nearly two hundred individuals (SCIA 2010a). In essence, the report said that hospitals serving Native Americans in the region had too few doctors and nurses to provide quality and timely health care to the patients, along with other financial and administrative issues that further impacted care.

The Dorgan Report was neither a revelation nor anything new to those who observe or live in Indian Country. IHS facilities have often lacked sufficient staff to effectively service the local population. As previously noted, funding has never matched demand and the service itself has often seemed a low governmental priority. The IHS has continually struggled to recruit quality doctors and well-trained nurses to serve at facilities in rural areas and without high salaries or prestige (Reed 2018). They have resorted to hiring people who would fail a typical background check. This practice was exposed in 2019 and 2020 when the *Wall Street Journal* published several investigative reports about health care on reservations (Weaver, Frosch, and Johnson 2019; Weaver, Frosch, and Schwartz 2019; *Wall Street Journal* 2020). These reports further showed that the IHS allowed questionable medical personnel who have engaged in criminal behavior and malpractice to continue to serve Native American communities, often for decades (Weaver, Frosch, and Schwartz 2019). The *Wall Street Journal* went further with their efforts by coproducing with PBS's *Frontline* an investigation called *Predator on the Reservation* (Johnson, Weaver, and Rosch 2019). This investigation revealed that Stanley Patrick Weber, a pediatrician convicted of sexually assaulting Native American boys in 2018, had been the subject of several whistle-blower complaints. Despite this pattern of behavior, Weber was protected by the agency and shuffled from one position to the next.

The Dorgan Report also revealed that some IHS facilities were at risk of losing Centers for Medicare and Medicaid Service (CMS) accreditation or certification due to deficiencies in management and service (SCIA 2010b, 5–6). CMS certification is a critical financial lynchpin in providing services as it enables IHS facilities to bill Medicare and Medicaid for services. IHS maintains a role as the "payer of last resort," meaning they only pay for services when all other options for payment, excluding out of a patient's pocket, have been exhausted. This coupled with the limited nature of federal appropriations to IHS makes third-party payments very important to the bottom line and the provision of services. Private insurance company (2 percent), Medicare (4 percent), and Medicaid (14 percent) payments constitute 20 percent of total IHS service program funding; Medicaid alone accounts for 70 percent of all third-party revenues (Boccuti, Swoope, and Artiga 2014, 7). As of 2017, over a quarter of non-elderly Native Americans and half of Native American children received health insurance through Medicaid, so the jeopardization of CMS status has major implications both for patient access to health care generally and for facilities' operational capacity (Artiga, Ubri, and Foutz 2017, 1). After the Dorgan Report's release, an article in *Indian Country Today* succinctly described its findings as "damning" and "horror-filled" (Capriccioso 2018).

QUENTIN N. BURDICK MEMORIAL HEALTH CARE FACILITY

In hearings connected to the release of the Dorgan Report, Chairman Dorgan provided an example he described as "horrendous" involving a nurse at Quentin N. Burdick Memorial Health Care Facility in Belcourt, North Dakota (SCIA 2010b). While in the throes of her addiction, the employee had been stealing drugs from the pharmacy and was found to be treating patients while in an "impaired state" in multiple incidents over a fourteen-year period. These included a cesarean section procedure, during which the nurse's faculties were so compromised that she "could not properly place and hold retractors and hold the patient's skin in place for staples." Like dozens of other substandard and criminal employees, the nurse was not terminated for her performance while impaired or offered help with her addiction but rather moved to a "desk job" to reach the twenty years of service required for full retirement benefits.

This was not the only troubling incident at Burdick Memorial. The 2010 Senate investigation found that the hospital pharmacy had "experienced substantial losses or thefts of Schedule II drugs since 2003" including oxycodone, fentanyl, and hydromorphone (SCIA 2010b, 16–17). In 2010, the Drug Enforcement Administration indicated that over twelve thousand alprazolam, diazepam, and propoxyphen pills were missing due to employee theft, and according to an IHS consulting report, over forty-eight thousand hydrocodone tablets could not be accounted for at the facility (SCIA 2010b). The hydrocodone incident eventually resulted in the arrest and convictions of five people (HHS 2017, 1), including two Burdick Memorial pharmacy employees (HHS 2011). The pharmacy also was providing refills of Schedule II drugs, a violation of federal regulations that require a doctor to write a new prescription for patients to obtain additional drugs (SCIA 2010b, 16–17). Given that Native Americans face higher rates of substance dependence and abuse than any other ethnic group in the country, due in part to factors such as historical trauma and poverty, Burdick Memorial's practice put an already vulnerable population at even greater risk (Barker 2013, 59–61).

Problems with management, staffing, and accountability were common at Burdick Memorial. The Senate investigation found that the hospital employed providers working with expired licenses and certifications, and that many did not have the adequate skills or training for the healthcare areas in which they were providing services. After reviewing twenty-eight employee files, it was found that ten lacked the required professional licenses and registrations, and mandated background checks or education verification were not conducted for eight and fifteen employees, respectively (SCIA 2010b, 28). Over a five-year period, twenty-two individuals were placed on administrative leave with an average duration of six weeks (8–9), a remedy often used in addition to transfers and reassignments to address issues with employee misconduct or performance (5). Rarely was anyone fired outright.

The consequences of Burdick Memorial's incompetence across multiple domains of health-care provision have had devastating impacts on the lives of patients, families, and communities. One example is twenty-four-year-old Shiree Wilson, who died a week after giving birth to her son. According to court documents from the wrongful death suit Wilson's mother filed against the IHS and five Burdick Memorial health-care providers, preoperative blood work for Wilson's planned cesarean section showed a high white blood cell count (a potential indicator of infection), and she informed doctors of a persistent cough. Two days following the baby's delivery, Wilson was discharged without any follow-up tests, only to return to the emergency room five days later due to shortness of breath and increased coughing. Testing during the emergency room visit revealed high blood pressure, a heart murmur, what her records described as a "mildly enlarged" heart, a continued high white blood cell count, and fluid in her lungs. Wilson was diagnosed with bilateral atypical pneumonia, prescribed decongestants with antibiotics, and was released the same day. One day later, she died (*Fluhrer v. U.S. et al.* 2015a).

An autopsy concluded that Wilson had severe pulmonary congestion and edema, in addition to her heart being twice the normal weight for her body mass index. The lawsuit claimed that medical malpractice and negligence on the part of the system resulted in a preventable death, leaving a newborn baby without his mother and a young husband without his wife (*Fluhrer v. U.S. et al.* 2015a, 3–7). The suit was eventually settled out of court and dismissed (*Fluhrer v. U.S. et al.* 2015b). The tragic nature of Wilson's story and its implications for IHS care reverberate well beyond her particular case.

SIOUX SAN HOSPITAL

The Rapid City Indian Health Service Hospital, formerly known as Sioux San Hospital, is another facility identified as problematic (Walker 2019). Established in 1898 as the Rapid City Indian School, it originally served as one of the federal government's boarding schools aimed at "assimilating" Native American children into the culture and ways of white, Christian society (NewsCenter1 2019). Thousands of children were forcibly removed from their families and placed in these schools, where abuse was commonplace and cultural erasure was the objective under the motto "Let all that is Indian within you die" (Robinson 2015). This policy of "civilization" has been identified as a major cause of intergenerational trauma among Native Americans (Bissonette and Shebby 2017). Forty-four children are known to have died at the Sioux San site from malnutrition and neglect (NewsCenter1 2019). After the school's closure in 1933, it was reopened in 1939 as the Sioux Sanitarium, a tuberculosis hospital for Native Americans where many died prior to the discovery of streptomycin in 1943. With the closing of the sanitarium in the early 1960s, the recently established IHS converted it to a hospital (Conti 2017).

The Dorgan Report identified serious shortcomings at Sioux San, including medical doctors practicing with expired state licenses (SCIA 2010b, 28); inadequate auditing of narcotics, resulting in the theft or loss of controlled substances; and large numbers of employee grievances filed for issues including reprisal and retaliation (10–11). In a statement submitted to the Senate Committee on Indian Affairs in 2010, Dr. Steven Miller relayed the story of a twenty-one-year IHS employee who was "denied leave for her mother's funeral; denied leave for her own surgery; harassed for reporting substance abuse of IHS employees; denied compensatory time and overtime; and received a low rating for the first time in 21 years on her performance evaluation—likely in retaliation for these other issues" (SCIA 2010b). In a 2016 statement to the Senate committee, which was again investigating health-care failures, Rosebud Sioux Tribe member Sunny Colombe discussed the resignation of a pediatrician who had successfully treated her daughter for a major health issue after another IHS facility was unable to do so. She described this doctor as always providing "the best care IHS had to offer" and expressed her sadness for the community when the pediatrician told her that she "just couldn't do it anymore" with respect to working at Sioux San (SCIA 2016, 132). Management issues created conditions in which talent remains difficult to retain (19), and a lack of accountability continues to perpetuate incompetence within the IHS system (104). As one Sioux San patient told *Native Sun News*, "All we see is doctors coming and going" (Chasing Hawk 2011).

Within the IHS, administrative problems have repeatedly led to patient harm and even deaths. Carry Schumacher, who went to the Sioux San emergency room after a horse-riding accident, was treated with muscle relaxers and pain medication, despite having a broken back and collar bone—conditions subsequently found by a non-IHS hospital (Chasing Hawk 2011). Marilyn Gayton went to Sioux San emergency room for pain and was released after being given pain medication. Later, Gayton learned that she had actually suffered a heart attack and now had pancreatic damage. Sioux San diagnosed none of these issues (Chasing Hawk 2011).

Robyn Black Lance brought her six-month-old son to Sioux San when he was having difficulty breathing. Doctors did not take his medical history, which included a premature birth and previous respiratory issues, and told her that his symptoms were due to a cold. Twelve hours after being released, they returned to the hospital emergency room because the baby's condition had worsened. Due to capacity issues at Sioux San, they were diverted to Rapid City Regional Hospital for treatment. Black Lance says that this coincidental move saved her son's life. There he received the proper diagnosis of RSV (respiratory syncytial virus) and spent a week and a half in intensive care before recovering (Walker 2019).

In May 2016, CMS informed Sioux San of their intent to terminate the facility's participation in their programs following an unannounced inspection of the facility. It was the fourth IHS hospital in two years to lose CMS certification (Associated Press 2016). According to the notification letter sent to hospital administrators, CMS found that the conditions at Sioux San "substantially limit the hospital's capacity to render adequate care" (CMS 2016) due to inadequate medical screening examinations to assess the presence of an emergency medical condition, placing patients in "immediate jeopardy" (Energy and Commerce 2016). CMS concluded that "these deficiencies are so serious that they constitute an immediate and serious threat to the health and safety of any individual who comes to your hospital to receive emergency services" (CMS 2016). The IHS closed the emergency room and inpatient services at Sioux San in September 2016 (Frosch 2017). While originally described as a temporary measure, the closures were subsequently made permanent. Only urgent care and outpatient services were maintained, exacerbating healthcare access issues in addition to concerns about the quality of care received by IHS patients (Walker 2019).

BETTER OUTCOMES IN A NEW FUTURE?

Both the 2010 Dorgan Report and the 2016 Senate hearing highlighted the continued "deficiencies in management, employee accountability, financial integrity, and oversight" within the IHS, which were allowed to persist over time and at great human cost (SCIA 2010b). While much of the government's focus has been on the Great Plains area, the problems with health care are more widespread in Indian Country (SCIA 2016, 4). Considering the federal government's failure to carry out its treaty and trust obligations with respect to providing health care via the IHS, tribes have increasingly taken control over the provision of health services as well as the management of facilities and hospitals, using the provisions of the ISDEAA of 1975. This marks a new and notable turn in the struggle for self-determination and local decision-making among Native Americans. Sioux San and Burdick Memorial demonstrate the long-standing inadequacies of the IHS as a service provider. However, because of the IS-DEAA and an evolution of federal-tribal relationships in recent years, the IHS has become more successful as a health-care facilitator. The evolution of the federal government's self-governance policy with respect to Native Americans has resulted in over 50 percent of all federal Indian programs being carried out by tribes rather than federal agencies (Strommer and Osborne 2014).

Indeed, the ISDEAA arose as a response to the self-determination movement of the 1960s and 1970s. It gives Title I federally recognized tribes or tribal organizations a combination of options where they can 1) continue to receive health-care services from IHS, 2) assume the responsibility for health care via funding agreements and self-governance compacts to receive funds from IHS, or 3) fund the establishment of their own health-care services or augment what is offered via IHS (IHS 2016). Option 2 allows tribes to invoke either Title I of the ISDEAA, which involves contracting for services (called Self-Determination Contracting), or Title V, which involves compacting for services (called Self-Governance Compacting) (IHS, n.d.). The ISDEAA's 638 "contracting" or "compacting" provisions (named after the numerical title of the IS-DEAA itself, Public Law 93–638) require the operation of any federal program, function, service, or activity (called PFSAs) to be transferred to tribes upon a formal request from the tribe (Herman and Fei, n.d.). This transfer is outlined in a contract often referred to as a "638 contract." Tribes may also form a "638 compact" over a federal PFSA with the federal government to co-operate the PFSA, which may have financial or administrative advantages for the tribe. "638ing" allows for federal monies that would have been directed to IHS facilities to be redirected to tribes so that they may organize and run the facility locally or have significantly more authority over how the funds are spent or how the facilities are run under a compact. Though it can be a costly, difficult, and controversial undertaking, 638ing provides an alternative to health care that is solely managed by the IHS (Giago Davies 2019; Ecoffey 2019).

With contract funding agreements and self-governance compacts, health care can now be a matter managed locally in a way that is best for the tribe. As of July 2016, the IHS and tribes have negotiated 90 self-governance compacts, funded through 115 agreements with over 350 federally recognized tribes (IHS 2016). Programs such as the Nuka System of Care in Southcentral Alaska and the efforts of the Reno-Sparks Indian Colony in Nevada are models of successful self-determination programs with various levels of IHS cooperation. Following decades of an unacceptable status quo, even Sioux San has recently transitioned to majority-tribal operation and management by the Great Plains Tribal Leaders' Health Board, a cooperative organization with representation from eighteen tribes in the region (Walker 2019). The transition has not been without controversy, as some in the local community are concerned that the new leadership is not up to the task of managing the facility and providing life and death care to thousands of Native Americans in the region (Giago 2019). At the time of this writing, Burdick Memorial remains under the sole control of the IHS.

The evolution of federal policy regarding self-determination has been key to tribes moving out of the long shadow of decades of inadequate federal funding and poor administration of programs for Native Americans. Since the passage of the ISDEAA in 1975, Native American tribal governments have had an increasingly larger role in providing and managing the health-care services that historically have been administered by the federal government. As in all things, a source of stable and secure funding is paramount to the better provision of health care for Native peoples. With the provisions of the IHCIA made permanent in 2010, and the contract and compact provisions of the ISDEAA in force, Native American tribes throughout the United States finally have a mechanism to circumvent long-standing federal dysfunction and work toward improving the nature and quality of local health outcomes.

REFERENCES

Adakai, Monique, Michelle Sandoval-Rosario, Fang Xu, Teresa Aseret-Manygoats, Michael Allison, Kurt Greenlund, and Kamil Barbour. 2018. "Health Disparities Among American Indians/Alaska Natives—Arizona, 2017." *Morbidity and Mortality Weekly Report* 67, no. 47: 1314–18. https://www.cdc.gov/mmwr /volumes/67/wr/mm6747a4.htm.

AICC (American Indian Chicago Conference). 1961. *Declaration of Indian Purpose: The Voice of the American Indian; Proceedings of the American Indian Chicago Conference (University of Chicago, Jun 13–20, 1961)*. Washington, D.C.: U.S. Department of Health Education, and Welfare, Office of Education. https:// files.eric.ed.gov/fulltext/ED030518.pdf.

Artiga, Samantha, Petry Ubri, and Julia Foutz. 2017. *Medicaid and American Indians and Alaska Natives.* San Francisco: Henry J. Kaiser Family Foundation, September 2017. http://files.kff.org/attachment/issue-brief-medicaid-and -american-indians-and-alaska-natives.

Associated Press. 2016. "Indian Health Service Facility Faulted for Treatment of 6-Month-Old." Indianz.com, May 24, 2016. https://www.indianz.com/News /2016/05/24/indian-health-service-facility-cited-for.asp.

Barker, Tammy R. 2013. "The Psychological Impact of Historical Trauma on the Native American People." Master's thesis, Regis University. *https://epublica-tions.regis.edu/theses/218/.*

Bissonette, Terri, and Susan Shebby. 2017. "Trauma-Informed School Practices: The Value of Culture and Community in Efforts to Reduce the Effects of Generational Trauma." American Psychological Association, Children Youth and Families News, December 2017. https://www.apa.org/pi/families/resources /newsletter/2017/12/generational-trauma.

Blansett, Kent. 2018. *A Journey to Freedom: Richard Oakes, Alcatraz, and the Red Power Movement.* New Haven, CT: Yale University Press.

Boccuti, Cristina, Christina Swoope, and Samantha Artiga. 2014. *The Role of Medicare and the Indian Health Service for American Indians and Alaska Natives: Health, Access and Coverage.* San Francisco: Henry J. Kaiser Family Foundation, December 2014. http://files.kff.org/attachment/report-the-role-of-medi care-and-the-indian-health-service-for-american-indians-and-alaska-natives -health-access-and-coverage.

Breiding, Matthew, J. Chen, and Michelle Black. 2014. *Intimate Partner Violence in the United States 2010.* Atlanta: National Center for Injury Prevention and Control/Centers for Disease Control and Prevention, February 2014. https:// www.cdc.gov/violenceprevention/pdf/cdc_nisvs_ipv_report_2013_v17_single _a.pdf.

Capriccioso, Rob. 2018. "Dorgan Releases Damning IHS Report." *Indian Country Today,* September 13, 2018. https://indiancountrytoday.com/archive/dorgan -releases-damning- ihs-report.

Chasing Hawk, Ernestine. 2011. "IHS Criticized for Service in South Dakota." *Native Sun News* (reposted on Indianz.com), May 25, 2011. https://www.indianz .com/News/2011/001723.asp.

Cherokee Nation. 2023. "History." Last updated June 9, 2023. https://www.cher okee.org/about-the-nation/history/.

CMS (Centers for Medicare and Medicaid Service). 2016. "23 Day Notice of Intent to Terminate Medicare Provider Agreement (May 23, 2016)." https:// www.indianz.com/News/2016/05/23/cmssiouxsan052316.pdf.

Conti, Kibbe. 2017. "The History of Sioux Sanitarium as a Segregated Tuberculosis Hospital." *Rapid City Journal*, May 4, 2017. https://issuu.com/rapidcity journal/docs/siouxsantab_fullproof.

CRS (Congressional Research Service). 2014. *The Indian Health Care Improvement Act Reauthorization and Extension as Enacted by the ACA: Detailed Summary and Timeline*. CRS Report R41630. Washington, D.C.: Congressional Research Service, updated January 3, 2014. https://crsreports.congress.gov/pro duct/pdf/R/R41630.

DeJong, David H. 2015. *American Indian Treaties: A Guide to Ratified and Unratified Colonial, United States, State, Foreign, and Intertribal Treaties and Agreements, 1607–1911*. Salt Lake City: University of Utah Press.

Ecoffey, Brandon. 2019. "Sioux San Run by OST and CRST." *Lakota Times*, June 13, 2019. https://www.lakotatimes.com/articles/sioux-san-run-by-ost -and-crst/.

Energy and Commerce (U.S. House of Representatives Committee on Energy and Commerce). 2016. "Letter to Mary L. Smith, Principal Deputy Director, Indian Health Service from Ranking Member Frank Pallone, Jr. (August 4, 2016)." https://energycommerce.house.gov/sites/democrats.energycommerce .house.gov/files/documents/IHS%20Smith%20IHS%20Hospitals%20Letter %202016%208%204.pdf.

Frieden, Joyce. 2020. "Native Americans Need More Funding to Battle COVID-19, Lawmakers Told." *MedPage Today*, June 12, 2020. https://www.medpagetoday .com/infectiousdisease/covid19/87032.

Frosch, Dan. 2017. "Indian Health Service to End Some Care at South Dakota Hospital." *Wall Street Journal*, July 28, 2017. https://www.wsj.com/arti cles/indian-health-service-to-close-more-services-at-south-dakota-hospital -1501279019.

GAO (U.S. Government Accountability Office). 2018. "Indian Health Service: Agency Faces Ongoing Challenges Filling Provider Vacancies." https://www .gao.gov/products/GAO-18-580.

Giago, Tim. 2019. "A Matter of Life and Death at Indian Health Service Hospital." *Indianz.com*, September 23, 2019. https://www.indianz.com/News/2019 /09/23/tim-giago-a-matter-of-life-and-death-at.asp.

Giago Davies, James. 2019. "Lawsuit Targets Tribal Takeover of IHS Hospital." *Native Sun News* (reposted on Indianz.com), August 14, 2019. https://www .indianz.com/News/2019/08/14/native-sun-news-today-lawsuit-targets-tr.asp.

Herman, Bob, and Fan Fei. n.d. "Taking Matters into Their Own Hands." *Modern Healthcare*, accessed May 12, 2021. www.modernhealthcare.com/reports /wounded-care/four.html.

HHS (U.S. Department of Health and Human Services). 2011. "Spotlight On . . .
Indian Health Service." Office of Inspector General. https://oig.hhs.gov/reports
-and-publications/archives/spotlight/2011/ihs.asp.

HHS (U.S. Department of Health and Human Services). 2017. *Two Indian Health
Service Hospitals Had System Security and Physical Controls for Prescription Drug
and Opioid Dispensing but Could Still Improve Controls*. Report No. A-18-
16-30540. Washington, D.C.: Office of Inspector General, November 2017.
https://oig.hhs.gov/oas/reports/region18/181630540.pdf.

IHS (Indian Health Service). 1985. *Indian Health Service: A Comprehensive Health
Care Program for American Indians and Alaska Natives*. Rockville, MD: Indian
Health Service. https://files.eric.ed.gov/fulltext/ED262940.pdf.

IHS (Indian Health Service). 2010. "Indian Health Care Improvement Act Made
Permanent" https://www.ihs.gov/newsroom/pressreleases/2010pressreleases
/indianhealthcareimprovementactmadepermanent/.

IHS (Indian Health Service). 2015. *Trends in Indian Health: 2014 Edition*. Rockville, MD: Indian Health Service, Division of Program Statistics, March 2015.
https://www.ihs.gov/sites/dps/themes/responsive2017/display_objects/docu
ments/Trends2014Book508.pdf.

IHS (Indian Health Service). 2016. "Tribal Self-Governance." https://www.ihs
.gov/newsroom/index.cfm/factsheets/tribalselfgovernance/.

IHS (Indian Health Service). 2020. "IHS Profile." https://www.ihs.gov/news
room/factsheets/ihsprofile/.

IHS (Indian Health Service). n.d. "Title I." Accessed May 26, 2021. https://www
.ihs.gov/odsct/title1/.

Indianz.com. 2015. "Yvette Roubideaux to Leave Obama Administration After
Six Years." Indianz.Com, June 2, 2015. https://www.indianz.com/News/2015
/017700.asp.

Johnson, Gabe, Christopher Weaver, and Dan Rosch, producers. *Frontline*. Season 2019, episode 7, "Predator on the Reservation." Aired February 12, 2019,
on PBS. https://www.pbs.org/wgbh/frontline/documentary/predator-on-the
-reservation/.

Jones, David S. 2006. "The Persistence of American Indian Health Disparities."
American Journal of Public Health 96 , no. 12 (December): 2122–34. https://doi
.org/10.2105%2FAJPH.2004.054262.

Kuschell-Haworth, Holly T. 2010. "A History of Federal Indian Health Care."
University of Dayton School of Law, Institute on Race, Health Care and the
Law. https://academic.udayton.edu/health/02organ/Indian03.htm.

Landry, Alysa. 2016. "Richard M. Nixon: 'Self-Determination Without Termination.'" *Indian Country Today*, September 13, 2016. https://indiancountrytoday

.com/archive/richard-m-nixon-self-determination-without-termination-K
-BgPAyGZ0GAkIY3OyS8-A.

Lawrence, Jane. 2000. "The Indian Health Service and the Sterilization of Native American Women." *American Indian Quarterly* 24, no. 3: 400–419. http://www
.jstor.org/stable/1185911.

Moorman, Lewis J. 1949. "Health of the Navajo-Hopi Indians: General Report of the American Medical Association Team." *Journal of the American Medical Association* 139, no. 6: 370–76. https://doi.org/10.1001/jama.1949.72900230001007.

Meriam, Lewis. 1928. *The Problem of Indian Administration*. Washington, D.C.: Brookings Institution. https://files.eric.ed.gov/fulltext/ED087573.pdf.

NewsCenter1. 2019. "Moving on from Tragedy, More Than 100 Years After Children Died at Rapid City Indian Boarding School." October 6, 2019. https://
www.newscenter1.tv/moving-on-from-tragedy-more-than-100-years-after
-children-died-at-rapid-city-indian-boarding-school/.

Nighthorse Campbell, Ben. 2007. "Opening Keynote Address: Activating Indians into National Politics." In *American Indian Nations: Yesterday, Today, and Tomorrow*, edited by George P. Horse Capture, Duane Champagne, and Chandler C. Jackson, 1–6. Lanham, MD: Altamira Press.

NLM (U.S. National Library of Medicine). 2012. "'If You Knew the Conditions . . .': Health Care to Native Americans." https://www.nlm.nih.gov/exhi
bition/if_you_knew/ifyouknew_06.html.

Pearson, J. Diane. 2003. "Lewis Cass and the Politics of Disease: The Indian Vaccination Act of 1832." *Wicazo Sa Review* 18, 2: 9–35. http://www.jstor.org
/stable/1409535.

Reed, Tina. 2018. "GAO: Indian Health Service Continues to Struggle Filling Provider Vacancies." *Fierce Healthcare*, August 17, 2018. https://www.fierce
healthcare.com/hospitals-health-systems/gao-indian-health-services-facing
-ongoing-challenges-filling-provider.

Reinhardt, Akim D. 2007. *Ruling Pine Ridge: Oglala Lakota Politics from the IRA to Wounded Knee*. Lubbock: Texas Tech University Press.

Rhoades, Everett R. 2009. "The Indian Health Services and Traditional Indian Medicine." *American Medical Association Journal of Ethics* 11, no. 10: 793–98. https://journalofethics.ama-assn.org/article/indian-health-service-and-tradi
tional-indian-medicine/2009-10.

Rhoades, Everett R., Anthony J. D'Angelo, and Ward B. Hurlburt. 1987. "The Indian Health Service Record of Achievement." *Public Health Reports (1974–)* 102, no. 4: 356–60. https://www.jstor.org/stable/4628165.

Rhoades, Everett R., Luana L. Reyes, and George D. Buzzard. 1987. "The Organization of Health Services for Indian People." *Public Health Reports (1974–)* 102, no. 4: 352–56. https://www.jstor.org/stable/4628164.

Rhoades, Everett R., and Dorothy A. Rhoades. 2014. "The Public Health Foundation of Health Services for American Indians and Alaska Natives." *American Journal of Public Health* 104, no. S3: 278–85. https://doi.org/10.2105/AJPH .2013.301767.

Rife, James P., and Alan J. Dellapenna. 2009. *Caring and Curing: A History of the Indian Health Service.* Cheltenham, MD: PHS Commissioned Officers Foundation for the Advancement of Public Health.

Robinson, Antoinette. 2015. "'Let All That Is Indian Within You Die'— Recognizing America's Brutal Legacy with Native American Families." *Rise Magazine,* September 1, 2015. https://www.risemagazine.org/2015/09/let-all -that-is-indian-within-you-die/.

Schroedel, Jean Reith. 2020. *Voting in Indian Country: The View from the Trenches.* Philadelphia: University of Pennsylvania Press.

SCIA (U.S. Senate Committee on Indian Affairs). 2010a. "Dorgan: Investigation Shows Indian Health Service in Aberdeen Area is in a 'Chronic State of Crisis.'" Press release. December 29, 2010. https://www.indian.senate.gov/news /press-release/dorgan-investigation-shows-indian-health-service-aberdeen -area-chronic-state.

SCIA (U.S. Senate Committee on Indian Affairs). 2010b. *In Critical Condition: The Urgent Need to Reform the Indian Health Service's Aberdeen Area.* Washington, D.C.: U.S. Senate, December 28, 2010. https://www.indian.senate .gov/sites/default/files/upload/files/ChairmansReportInCriticalCondition 122810.pdf.

SCIA (U.S. Senate Committee on Indian Affairs). 2016. *Reexamining the Substandard Quality of Indian Health Care in the Great Plains: Hearing Before the Committee on Indian Affairs of the United States Senate.* 114th Congress, February 3, 2016. https://www.govinfo.gov/content/pkg/CHRG-114shrg21662 /html/CHRG-114shrg21662.htm.

Shelton, Brett Lee. 2004. *Legal and Historical Roots of Health Care for American Indians and Alaska Natives in the United States.* San Francisco: Henry J. Kaiser Family Foundation, February 2004. https://www.kff.org/wp-content/uploads /2013/01/legal-and-historical-roots-of-health-care-for-american-indians-and -alaska-natives-in-the-united-states.pdf.

Smith, Paul Chaat, and Robert Allen Warrior. 1996. *Like a Hurricane: The Indian Movement from Alcatraz to Wounded Knee.* New York: New Press.

St. J. Perrott, George, and Margaret D. West. 1957. "Health Services for American Indians." *Public Health Reports (1896–1970)* 72, no. 7: 565–70. https://doi.org /10.2307/4589827.

Strommer, Geoffrey D., and Stephen D. Osborne. 2014. "The History, Status, and Future of Tribal Self-Governance Under the Indian Self-Determination and

Education Assistance Act." *American Indian Law Review* 39, no. 1. https://digitalcommons.law.ou.edu/ailr/vol39/iss1/1/.

Tjaden, Patricia, and Nancy Thoennes. 1998. *The Prevalence, Incidence, and Consequences of Violence Against Women: Findings from the National Violence Survey Against Women*. Washington, D.C.: National Institute of Justice and Centers for Disease Control and Prevention, November 1998. https://www.ojp.gov/pdffiles/172837.pdf.

USCCR (U.S. Commission on Civil Rights). 2018. *Broken Promises: Continuing Federal Funding Shortfall for Native Americans*. Washington, D.C.: U.S. Commission on Civil Rights, December 2018. https://www.usccr.gov/pubs/2018/12-20-Broken-Promises.pdf.

Walker, Mark. 2019. "Fed Up with Deaths, Native Americans Want to Run Their Own Health Care." *New York Times*, October 15, 2019. https://www.nytimes.com/2019/10/15/us/politics/native-americans-health-care.html.

Wall Street Journal. 2020. "Forsaken by the Indian Health Service." January 16, 2020. https://www.wsj.com/articles/forsaken-by-the-indian-health-service-11579196871.

Warne, Donald, and Linda Bane Frizzell. 2014. "American Indian Health Policy: Historical Trends and Contemporary Issues." *American Journal of Public Health* 104, no. S3 (June): S263–67. https://doi.org/10.2105/AJPH.2013.301682.

Weaver, Christopher, Dan Frosch, and Gabe Johnson. 2019. "A Pedophile Doctor Drew Suspicions for 21 Years. No One Stopped Him." *Wall Street Journal*, February 8, 2019. https://www.wsj.com/articles/a-pedophile-doctor-drew-suspicions-for-21-years-no-one-stopped-him-11549639961?mod=article_inline.

Wilkins, David E., and Heidi K. Stark. 2011. *American Indian Politics and the American Political System*. 3rd ed. Lanham, MD: Rowman & Littlefield.

LEGAL RESOURCES

Act to Establish the Home Department, Ch. 108, § 1, 9 Stat. 395 (1849)

Affordable Care Act, Pub. L. No. 111–148, 124 Stat. 119 (2010)

Cherokee Nation v. Georgia, 30 U.S. 1 (1831)

Fluhrer v. United States et al. 2015a, case no. 4:15-cv-00165, dismissed in 8th. Cir. Case filing can be accessed at https://www.indianz.com/News/2016/04/11/fluhrervus.pdf.

Fluhrer v. United States et al. 2015b, case no. 4:15-cv-00165, dismissed in 8th. Cir. Case documents can be accessed at https://www.pacermonitor.com/case/9951605/Fluhrer_v_United_States_of_America_et_al.

Indian Health Care Improvement Act, S. 522, 94th Congress (1976)

Indian Reorganization Act, 25 U.S.C. Ch. 14, Subch. 5 § 461 et seq. (1975)

Indian Sanitation Facilities Act, Pub. L. No. 86–121, 73 Stat. 267 (1959)

Indian Self-Determination and Education Assistance Act, Pub. L. No. 93–68, 88 Stat. 2203 (1975)

Indian Vaccination Act, H.R. 526, 22nd Cong. (1832)

Johnson-O'Malley Act, Pub. L. No. 115–404, 132 Stat. 5349 (1934)

Johnson v. M'Intosh, 21 U.S. 543 (1823)

Snyder Act, Pub. L. No. 67–85, 42 Stat. 208 (1921)

Tribal Self-Governance Act, H.R. 3508, 103rd Congress (1994)

Worcester v. Georgia, 31 U.S. (6 Pet.) 515 (1832)

3

THE PURSUIT OF WELLNESS AND DECOLONIZATION THROUGH CENTERING STORIES OF POST-9/11 NATIVE VETERANS

LEOLA TSINNAJINNIE PAQUIN

JOSEPH H. SUINA (2005) STATES, "The true meaning of sovereignty is that we still carry the spirit of our ancestors in our hearts." Indigenous Peoples of the twenty-first century continue to be lifted by the spirit of our ancestors while remaining resilient through the continuing oppressive forces of colonization in the forms of war, health disparities, deepening social inequalities, racialization and dehumanization, policies designed to strip Native nations and communities of self-determination, capitalism-driven resource extraction, and climate change. Fighting for Indigenous health and justice has never been more critical. It is up to Indigenous Peoples and our relatives to find new dimensions to our capacity to reclaim, protect, and sustain our well-being. This chapter explores a question that led to a study I completed in 2011: What does it mean to pursue wellness and decolonization as a Native veteran of the post-9/11 Bush era? A key consideration when conducting this research was that rethinking participation in American warfare should not be seen as disrespectful to our Native veteran populations and their families who consider their military service to be an honor and an active decision to protect the ancestral homeland. This scholarship honors the value of their lives and our collective humanity for the future.

In terms of wellness and decolonization, many of the participants spoke to the following: 1) trying to find well-being before, during, and after their service; 2) wanting to grow their knowledge in life through service; and 3) critiquing systems of oppression as they pertain to the military. In situating these reflections, I defined wellness as spiritual connectedness, health of mind, positive sense of physical capacity, being of service, building knowledge, and financial security in relation to family, community, and Indigenous land. This differs from non-Indigenous concepts of wellness that focus on the body and/or the mind but not on the relationships between the individual and the larger world. Indigenous wellness, among other things, focuses on interconnectedness, spirituality, and community. In the most direct sense, to have "health and wellness" is to have life, while war is trauma leading to the loss of body, land, ways of being, and inner peace.

THE STUDY

The overall purpose of the study, "Examining the Indigenous Relationship Between Education and the United States Military from 2001–2009" (Tsinnajinnie 2011), was to examine Native American service in the U.S. military from September 11, 2001, to January 2009 in order to point out the impacts of military service on Indigenous wellness, as such service is designed to maintain the U.S. social hierarchy domestically and globally through warfare.[1] I focused on this time frame because it was the period during which (white, wealthy) Republican George W. Bush was U.S. president. This is the period in which the United States began to implement the war on terror through invasions into Iraq and Afghanistan.

The study was based on both phenomenological and Indigenous methodology. The theoretical framework was structured primarily by Tribal Critical Race Theory (TribalCrit) and decolonization concepts. Bryan Brayboy, who developed TribalCrit, states that being able to not only listen to stories but to hear them is central to this framework. He shares, "Stories often are the guardians of cumulative knowledges that hold a place in the psyches of the group members, memories of tradition, and reflections of power. Hearers ultimately understand the nuances in stories and recognize that the onus for hearing is placed on the hearer rather

---

1. All study participant quotes included in this essay are from interviews conducted in 2011.

than the speaker for delivering a clearly articulated message. Additionally, one must be able to feel the stories. You tell them, hear them, and feel them—establishing a strong place for empathy and for 'getting it'" (Brayboy 2005, 440).

Eighteen participants were interviewed, one participant engaged in a presentation on the topic, and three participants contributed surveys alone. There were twenty-two participants overall, with ten identified as primary participants who experienced the phenomenon of entering or reenlisting in the military since September 11, 2001. The majority of the participants were from Native tribes of the Southwest. The major finding was that education was a motivating force for Native veterans in all aspects of their experience. They either considered military service as a component of their education and/or utilized the benefits earned in the military to complete college degrees.

This motivation for their enlistment needs to be contextualized by the physical and mental risks they were accepting.

THE IMPACTS OF WAR ON SERVING MEMBERS AND VETERANS

According to a congressional report, of the 29,676 Operation Iraqi Freedom casualties from March 19, 2003, to April 5, 2008, 302 were American Indian or Alaska Native (Fischer, Klarman, and Oboroceanu 2008). The following list provides a further sampling of the injuries and loss of life from the events of September 11, 2001, through mid-2008. Based on a Congressional Research Service report updated on May 14, 2008, Fischer, Klarman, and Oboroceanu (2008) reported the following, in addition to the casualties mentioned above:

- Of 3,866 Operation Iraqi Freedom deaths from May 1, 2003 to April 5, 2008, 38 were American Indian or Alaska Native.
- Of 487 Operation Enduring Freedom deaths from October 7, 2001, to April 5, 2008, 7 were American Indian or Alaska Native.
- Of 1,914 Operation Enduring Freedom military wounded in action (no dates specified), 23 were American Indian or Alaska Native.

The following statistics provide data on the population of Native American war veterans, according to a demographic report from the National Center for Veterans Analysis and Statistics (2017). The numbers were not broken down by tribe and represent various self-reports of Native identification. While these statistics are not reflective of the number of veterans at the time of the study, due to attrition, they were the best available at the time of writing.

- 1,470 veterans of World War II
- 5,725 veterans of the Korean conflict
- 44,911 veterans of the Vietnam era
- 24,884 veterans of the Gulf War (August 199–August 2001)
- 33,538 veterans of the Gulf War (September 2001 to 2017)

According to Korshak, Washington, and Birdwell, today American Indian and Alaska Native veterans suffer much poorer health outcomes than other veterans. About 74 percent of them use U.S. Department of Veterans Affairs (VA) health care and about 33 percent of them access mental health services through the VA. They "experience posttraumatic stress disorder (PTSD) at a greater rate than all other Veteran groups; AI/AN [American Indian and Alaska Native] Veterans have almost double the rate of PTSD as non-Hispanic white Veterans (20.5 percent versus 11.6 percent). A 2016 VA tribal consultation with all 567 federally recognized tribes identified treatment for PTSD and mental health as a top priority for Veterans in Indian Country" (Korshak, Washington, and Birdwell, n.d.).[2] The authors suggest that the disproportionate prevalence of PTSD suffered by Indigenous veterans may be rooted in "stress related to racial stereotypes" and compounded by barriers to care, socioeconomic status, and lack of culturally appropriate treatment facilities (Korshak, Washington, and Birdwell, n.d.).

Physical health issues are equally disparate. "AI/AN Veterans also experience chronic pain, especially low back and lower extremity pain, and are diagnosed with diabetes at higher rates than non-Hispanic white Veterans." The risks are especially high for women veterans, for whom

---

2. The number of federally recognized tribes as of this writing is 574 (see Schwartz 2023).

pregnancy may be complicated by hypertension or diabetes at "two times higher in AI/AN women than non-Hispanic white women" (Korshak, Washington, and Birdwell n. d.). Huyser et al. (2021, S69) report that Native veterans have a "high burden of functional disability," with 32 percent reporting some sort of physical limitation.

Clearly, along with the rest of the United States, Native nations are sacrificing the health and welfare of their youth, and their future, to war. Furthermore, these statistics speak to the unfortunate and extreme incidence of PTSD among Indigenous veterans. Yet, despite such statistics, many Native young people still consider military service as an opportunity.

The next section presents a few very small windows into powerful stories shared by Native veterans during the 2011 study, which are then considered within the context of U.S. conflicts in the twenty-first century. The chapter concludes with final considerations about the pursuit of wellness for Native veterans.

STORIES AND ANALYSIS

One study participant, Darren, explained the contempt he had for the Dixie Chicks (who have since renamed their band the Chicks), which stemmed from the comments made by lead singer Natalie Maines at a 2003 concert in London. Maines proclaimed the group was against the impending invasion of Iraq and was ashamed that President George W. Bush was from Texas. Darren, who is Diné, served in the U.S. Marine Corps from 2001 to 2005, and graduated from a university in 2011, said:

> The main singer, she made a big deal about the war and she talked against the war and she put down the president. Even though maybe, bless his heart, maybe the president was a jerk for sending us there but regardless you couldn't help the situation. Because it goes by a chain of command so . . . there's a hierarchy there that you have to respect. And then when someone tarnishes the reputation of the country by their liberalism. You know, it's very offensive, especially someone that doesn't even know what she's talking about. . . . But at the same time, you do understand that there's a protocol of freedom of speech. But . . . there's a certain time to say things. . . . You respect what people are going through. . . . She didn't respect the country's

space. And she didn't think about the young men and women that were fighting over there for her trench coats and her microphones.

Darren felt that to criticize the commander in chief was to criticize the military as a whole. Respect was a life lesson that Darren sought to live by.

Another participant, Jayson (Diné/Pueblo, who served in the U.S. Army from 2003 to 2009 and graduated from university in 2010), expressed his views on what it means to be Native versus a soldier.

I think there's people that have the warrior spirit in them. And I think that should be in them and I think they were born with that gift. And I think they were born with it as a blessing. But I don't think you use that to go make war on people. And I don't think you use that gift to go to another country and abuse it. I think you use that gift to learn the most you can out of it. And when people really do need defending or people really do need you to step up like in communities where you have meth going on or you have these little Native American gangs thinking they're all tough or stupid shit like that. Yeah, like, put your warrior spirit into action and do something about it. Like, don't go to Afghanistan and try solving the U.S. problem about oil . . . and so to me it's like I don't have nothing against the warrior spirit. I don't have nothing against a person that wants to use that, but I wish someone would put more thought into how they do it. Or not do it just because it pays money. And do it for a moral or a just reason.

He did not see the military as an outlet for the warrior spirit. Early on in our communication, Jayson told me that the military was no place for a Native person.

As a high school student, participant Vicente (Diné) refrained from taking the Armed Services Vocational Aptitude Battery (ASVAB) test so that he would not be visible to the U.S. military. He said, "I chose not to take the ASVAB. . . . I didn't want them to know what I knew." Vicente did not want to be recruited and share his knowledge and skills with them; he ultimately did not enlist, and graduated from college in 2010.

In these narratives, these men represent the beauty, pain, conflict, and hope of Native communities. This array of voices demonstrates the diversity of our people and the spirit of our ancestors.

The cost of Indigenous participation in the military in the twenty-first century, during a time of conflict, became apparent to Indian Country in 2003 when news spread that U.S. Army soldier Lori Piestewa was killed in Iraq—she is believed to be the first Native woman soldier killed in combat outside the United States (National Museum of the United States Army, n.d.). In June 2011, Celeste (Hopi/Hispanic), who began her service in the U.S. Army Reserve in 2007 and had just earned her master's degree the month prior to our meeting, responded to a question about which veterans she admired:

> Well of course Lori Piestewa. . . . I read a book called *I'm Still Standing[: From Captive U.S. Soldier to Free Citizen—My Journey Home]* by Shoshana Johnson and she tells that story from a different perspective. . . . I read it and kind of passed it around my unit so they could read it. But just reading that story and not really knowing, 'cause if you don't know about the military it's difficult to understand like what really happened. And then studying public administration and tribal administration and studying about politics and I did a couple of research papers on the invasion of Iraq. So just learning all of that and knowing what they were put through and . . . just the danger they were in . . . I don't know. I'm trying to find a nice way to put this, but . . . it was almost like they were sacrificed, you know what I mean? And when I think about her being the first Native American female killed in combat, I mean yeah, that's great but she didn't have to be there. She had two kids and, you know, every time I think about it, it just makes me, like, really emotional.

Celeste related to Lori as a Native, a mother, a fellow servicewoman, and someone who also experienced deployment in the same conflict in Iraq. As a survivor, Celeste was able to continue her education and her analysis of the situation she and those around her were in. Celeste, as well as two other mothers in this study, had to weigh the benefits and risks of reenlistment, including receiving military compensation versus trying to maintain a livelihood in civilian life. For Lori Piestewa, the choice to reenlist or exit was taken with her life. Celeste continued to reflect on the incident:

> It's stupid mistakes . . . people made and that's the part that really bothers me. . . . Yeah, it's sad because . . . She was active duty. She was a driver.

She was driving. It was just a wrong turn. You know and leaving behind her two kids. . . . I can't imagine. And although she's a hero, like, I really admire her. . . . I just felt so bad. I'm like, that would be awful. That would be so scary. And then to think that she could have possibly been saved or been alive, you know, and still have been injured. And they don't know the story and the government is covering up all these stories and not telling the truth. I'm like, okay you've already done this enough to our people. Like, at least be straight up and honest and tell, for her parents' sake her kids' sake . . . exactly what happened. Because they do that a lot. I mean . . . I experience it all the time. . . . So just thinking, just from what I studied . . . from the invasion is that the military really didn't have a plan. Like, they didn't have a sure plan and they had no idea what they were getting into. So they sent all these young men and women to a foreign country with not even some of the proper equipment to go there and fight this war. And a lot of people lost their lives for what cause? . . . And so I have a lot of mixed emotions about this war. But on the other hand, I have an obligation to my country because that's the decision I made.

Native America still mourns the loss of Lori Piestewa. For a young mother to decide the best way to help her children is to leave the reservation, risk her life, and serve in the military raises an obvious question: How voluntary is this institution?

Phillip, another research participant, served in the army for five years while taking a break from an elite private college where he could no longer afford to pay his tuition. He narrowly avoided the same fate as Lori—he was on the same path on the same mission as Lori on the day her envoy took the wrong turn that eventually led to an ambush and her death. He lives with this connection to her. After he told his story of survival, he brought up the racism that erupted in the movement to rename Squaw Peak in Phoenix, Arizona, to Piestewa Peak. He drew connections between Indigenous life, death, and the realities of Native representation in the United States. Again, like Celeste, Phillip is speaking to the loss of Indigenous life and contemplating the meaning of it in terms of how Natives are actually valued in the United States, both inside and outside the military.

Santa Ana Pueblo's Emilian Sanchez was killed in the same war four years later, in January of 2007 (Military Times, n.d.). He had followed the tradition of thousands of Natives before him and entered the U.S. military. When I asked Faren, a Pueblo participant in the study with a family legacy of military service, what helped him make his decision to enlist, he shared: "Actually, Emilian Sanchez . . . really sealed the deal for me. You know when he got killed? . . . That very next year, that day of my seventeenth birthday, I signed up." At the time of his interview, Faren was serving in the Marines but was not deployed in a country seeing combat action. While many of the participants were hesitant in accepting monetary compensation for their time or travel to meet with a researcher, Faren outright refused. My interpretation of the situation was that he was so driven by his ideals and what he represented that he could not accept money for something he felt was of service to another person. Furthermore, he could not pass on that money to his family because he was already able to give to them what he wished to provide. There was definitely a sense of honor from Faren, and from each person participating, which was evident in my observations of homes, schools, meetings, powwows, social media networking, friendships, and communities. Like Faren and other interviewees, these spaces demonstrated many elements of wellness as it was defined earlier: spiritual connectedness, health of mind, positive sense of physical capacity, being of service, building knowledge, and financial security in relation to family, community, and Indigenous land.

DECOLONIZING U.S. CONFLICTS IN THE TWENTY-FIRST CENTURY

There are countless stories to be told of family and friends who joined the military because of the educational opportunities either provided or promised. Structurally unequal privileges like financial wealth, political power, race, religion, sexual orientation, and family legacy play a key role in who has access to these opportunities. For example, the children of politicians and wealthy entrepreneurs usually do not have to join the military in order to have college prospects. Moreover, educational rewards are only available if servicepeople survive the war and meet all the requirements of the GI Bill. It is necessary, therefore, to critically examine the relationship between well-being and Native American enlistment in the U.S. military.

The political period of 2001 to 2009 in the United States was chiefly shaped by the fear of terrorism as a result of the September 11, 2001, attacks; U.S. engagement in a war opposed by the United Nations; and the Patriot Act. To understand this period, it is necessary to closely examine the conflicts in which the United States engaged: Operation Enduring Freedom and Operation Iraqi Freedom (Fischer, Klarman, and Oboroceanu 2008).

As demonstrated by the names given to the wars by the former commander in chief's administration, *freedom* was the rhetorical linchpin used to justify the military efforts of the United States. On September 20, 2001, George W. Bush planted the conceptual seed of fighting for freedom by stating, "Tonight we are a country awakened to danger and called to defend freedom. Our grief has turned to anger, and anger to resolution. Whether we bring our enemies to justice, or bring justice to our enemies, justice will be done" (Bush 2001). The societal cost of the war to U.S. citizens, along with the 4,237 U.S. military lives lost (as of January 2009), was an immeasurable catastrophe. Iraq suffered even greater losses: their estimated total deaths as of January 2009 included 8,890 Iraqi security forces members and over 44,434 Iraqi civilians (Iraq Coalition Casualty Count 2009). These numbers are likely serious underestimates and also do not speak to the trauma of the invasion or the destruction of land and daily ways of life. According to Iraq Body Count, a human security project, the documented civilian death count from violence ranged from 103,158 to 112,724 (Iraq Body Count 2011). In contrast, according to a study by the Watson Institute for International and Public Affairs at Brown University, "The biggest financial beneficiaries of the post-9/11 military spending surge have been major U.S.-based weapons contractors" (Hartung 2021, 5). Operation Iraqi Freedom was clearly a monetary win for American corporations and a devastation for many Iraqis who lost lives, resources, and ways of being. In essence, one could argue that this war did not focus on battles for freedom but battles for the maintenance of global economic, political, and social supremacy for the few with access to power and wealth.

Native scholar-activists have critiqued the Iraq War from a perspective of decolonization. Elizabeth Cook-Lynn argues that the twentieth-century wars in Iraq have paralleled the history of white-Indian conflict. She asserts, specifically:

Colonial tactics have remained fairly constant throughout history and they should be recognized today as strategies to diminish freedom for innocent and sovereign peoples. One of the aspects of this history that makes it crucial for all Americans to ponder is that certain political assumptions on the part of the United States reflected during the nineteenth and twentieth centuries are with us today. The foremost of these assumptions on the part of the United States are racial superiority felt by whites, the innocence of colonization felt by all capitalists, and the righteousness felt by all Christians—all assumptions that allow and encourage the United States to use its power to enforce its vision of itself as the indispensable democracy. (2007, 86)

At the time of this research, and today, the United States touts itself as a nation of freedom in which any person of any race or ethnicity may succeed, yet this runs counter to the Indigenous ideal of community well-being. White dominant society has continued to prevail, as indicated by economic and educational stratification reported by the U.S. Census Bureau (2008) closest to the time period of the 2011 study. American Indians and Alaska Natives were reported to have more than twice the ratio of people living below the poverty line than that of all residents combined. In terms of bachelor's degree attainment, 24 percent of the total population had college degrees while the number for Alaska Natives and American Indians was 11 percent.

The ultimate excuse for U.S. aggression and occupation has long been Christianity. From the European colonization of the Americas to Manifest Destiny to the invasion and occupation of Iraq, Christianity in practice as Christian nationalism has prevailed. The imposition of Christianity has essentially been a green light for the murder of Indigenous populations and the rape of their land. As a country that supposedly honors freedom of religion, the United States has a poor record of supporting *human rights*, both inside and outside its borders. Further evidence of Christian domination can be found in federal Indian law from the *Johnson v. M'Intosh* decision to supposedly protective federal legislation such as the American Indian Religious Freedom Act of 1978. For instance, according to Newcomb (2008), the Christian doctrine of discovery was adopted into U.S. law as a result of the *Johnson v. M'Intosh* case, which granted the power of dominion to the U.S. government over Indians.

This historical record should give little motivation for Native Americans to support the advancement of Christianity or capitalism through the use of the military, as is the current trend.

So why is it that Native Americans continue to serve in a military that engages in wars that do not appear to serve the interests of Native peoples or their lands? Again, in observing the revered treatment of veterans by many Native communities, there is a connection between warriorhood and service in U.S. military operations. In the Bush administration era, the Navajo Nation utilized a billboard near Window Rock, Arizona, with an image of what can be perceived as a traditional warrior turning into a police officer, to recruit young Navajo into service. This is an example of how Native American communities conceptualize and illustrate future pathways. In educational settings, sociocultural knowledge steers students' understanding of the importance of education, career, and family goals as they relate to their schooling (Miller and Brickman 2004). Research also suggests that when Native students are able to directly associate school tasks with perceptions of the future, they are motivated to strive toward academic achievements (Brickman, McInerney, and Martin 2009). The more sociocultural knowledge they absorb, from as many angles as possible, the more opportunity Indigenous youth have to invest their energies (academic or not) into futures that will support their well-being.

Michael Yellow Bird argued for Native American resistance to participating in the Iraq War (2007) and made a call for protests in his widely distributed Brown Paper (2012). He suggested that Native nations think critically about how our culture informs our decisions regarding participation in or refusal of war: "Maybe, just maybe, if we act using our traditional Indigenous forms of morality that value truth, intelligence, honesty, life, and dignity—and refuse to be a [*sic*] enabler to the U.S. addiction to greed, war, power, and colonization—we can help it overcome its unhealthy, destructive obsession for war, conquest, and killing of others" (Yellow Bird 2006). Yellow Bird provides a clear distinction between Indigenous values and the values that have driven the United States to war. In marking this distinction, he opens a dialogue that reconsiders Indigenous militarization. What does Indigenous warriorhood truly mean to our communities in this day?

It is interesting that many Native Americans envision warriorhood as a spirit in an intellectual battlefield where Indigenous people become warriors of education. They believe that the Indigenization of educational pathways through curriculum, pedagogy, community empowerment, and leadership is absolutely necessary if we are to resist, prevent, and overcome colonization. By creating resistance toward colonization, we are preserving lives, honoring families, saving our bodies, protecting mental well-being, and channeling energies into becoming educational warriors (Pewewardy 2005).

Further articulating the need to view Operation Iraqi Freedom from a critical Indigenous perspective, Yellow Bird (2006) describes the relationship between U.S. war efforts and Native American involvement:

> We must no longer allow our nations to remain in the fog of war, participating in the U.S. continued colonization and destruction of the world. What this country has done—and continues to do—to the Iraqi people is unconscionable and must stop. The U.S.-led war in Iraq is wrong, immoral, illegal, unjust, a lie; it is about profiteering for a very small, corrupt, elite sector of the U.S. population. Our people, many of whom occupy some of the lowest levels of decision-making in the U.S. military, are considered expendable and are being used for cannon fodder so that the rich, especially in the United States, can become richer.

Michael Yellow Bird's call to action (see also Yellow Bird 2012) and other efforts to mobilize a nonviolent intellectual path for Native warriorhood are significant signs that the spirit of decolonization is growing a dialogue at the intersection of education, Indigenous well-being, and the U.S. armed forces. While Yellow Bird's critique of the military clearly expresses his individual opposition to the war, this discussion repeatedly becomes clouded when examining Native Americans in the military from a broader perspective. In other words, individuals have spoken to the need to reconsider Native American participation in the military, but there has yet to be a majority collective voice discouraging enlistment. Social and cultural paradigms could hold the answer.

The Native American population at large is portrayed in the media as being patriotic and supportive of the military due to both the opportunities the system offers and to what has been coined the "warrior tradition" in Native society. A *St. Louis Post-Dispatch* article describes a scene in which Native American veterans were honored at a powwow:

Two dozen military veterans enter the powwow grounds to the sound of a drum's rhythmic thump and the chants of songs passed down from their ancestors. . . . They dance clockwise, a slow stutter step on lush grass, as sunlight dapples through the surrounding forest. Several are squeezed into old dress uniforms or camouflage fatigues. Many sport caps from which an eagle feather dangles; graying ponytails spill out the backs. A few wear traditional headdresses, breechcloths and leggings. . . . Above them, suspended from two soaring pines, a large American flag ripples in the breeze. (O'Connor and Crowe 2008)

This mainstream newspaper continues to paint the image of the honorable warrior tradition by quoting seventeen-year-old Vince Crow. "'It's a way to show pride,' Vince says. 'Pride for your family. Pride for your heritage. Pride for your nation. It just kind of goes along with our ancestry. Instead of protecting a village, you're protecting a country.'" He was referenced again later in the article: "Vince, his hair shaved close, wears a colorful beaded choker. A medicine pouch filled with tobacco dangles from his neck. He says he grew up listening to the tales of forefathers who found honor in battle. 'It goes with our heritage,' he says. 'Warriors, you know?'" (O'Connor and Crowe 2008).

While the article does centralize the idea of the warrior tradition as being a major factor in why Native Americans have the highest per capita record of military service, it does not mention poor physical and mental health, poverty, and lack of opportunity in hometowns. Although this is only one example of how Native American military service has been portrayed and/or understood, it is fairly representative of the general perception that Native American communities have of veterans. As indicated in the article, the status of Native veterans is especially visible when they are recognized in the grand entry at powwows. According to the Native-owned website PowWows.com (n.d.),

During the Grand Entry, everyone is asked to stand as the flags are brought into the arena. The flags carried generally include the U.S. flag, Tribal Flags, the POW Flag, and Eagle Staffs of various Native Nations present. These are usually carried by veterans. Native Americans hold the United States flag in an honored position despite the horrible treatment received from this country. The flag has a dual meaning. First, it is a way to remember all of the ancestors that fought against this country. It is also the symbol of the United States[, of] which Native Americans are now a part. The flag here also reminds people of those people who have fought for this country.

Not only are Native American veterans revered at powwow events, but they are widely recognized in many other facets of societal life. Veterans' names are recognized through displays in spaces such as Navajo Nation chapter houses. Native veteran organizations/conferences are supported by the community and tribes through monetary contributions and high rates of attendance. In celebrations or other events, Navajo code talkers are often invited as special guests of honor.

This raises the question of whether this representation of Native Americans as warriors supports the interests of the United States or Indigenous Peoples. CEHIP Incorporated (1996), in a report for the U.S. Department of Defense, describes Native American participation as being a form of twentieth-century warriorhood. They unmistakably name this relationship in their report:

As the 20th century comes to a close, there are nearly 190,000 Native American military veterans. It is well recognized that, historically, Native Americans have the highest record of service per capita when compared to other ethnic groups. The reasons behind this disproportionate contribution are complex and deeply rooted in traditional American Indian culture. In many respects, Native Americans are no different from others who volunteer for military service. They do, however, have distinctive cultural values which drive them to serve their country. One such value is their proud warrior tradition. . . . In part, the warrior tradition is a willingness to engage the enemy in battle. This characteristic has been clearly demonstrated by the courageous deeds of Native Americans in combat. However, the warrior tradition is best exemplified by the following qualities said to be inherent to most if not all Native American societies: strength, honor, pride, devotion, and wisdom. The qualities make a perfect fit with military tradition.

This representation is not supported completely by reality. For example, Apache Vietnam veteran Sam Ybarra became infamous for atrocious war crimes as a private in the Tiger Force commando unit and later died on his reservation while suffering from severe depression (Sallah and Weiss 2006). The cultural values the above report refers to, in Indigenous cultures, do not include killing, invading, and a lack of critical thinking.

Allowing the U.S. Department of Defense to make blanket connections between Native culture and service to the U.S. military is to allow the colonizer to further attack our sovereignty.

My argument can be summarized this way: The occupation of Iraq was controversial due to the casualties on all sides, which contrasted starkly with the monetary wealth obtained by profiteers of the war. Given these circumstances, and the United States' history of invasion and colonization, Native American participation in the military needs to be reconsidered in light of Indigenous nationhood. Examining ways in which social justice and the wellness of Indigenous communities can be achieved offers a key perspective on the subject.

CONCLUSION

As study participant Celeste expressed about enlistees' relationship to the U.S. military,

> The government's going to use you for their purposes and they're going to get everything they can. And this is what I always tell my soldiers, I'm like, "They're going to use you for everything you have. So why don't you use them for everything they have? Every benefit. Every dollar they can give you. You take advantage of that whether it's health care, whether it's monetary, gifts, or . . . education benefits. I mean, use that to the max. Give your kids your benefits or, you know, something." I'm like, "Because they will take everything they can from you." . . . I try not to be too pessimistic about that, but sometimes that's just how it is.

Indigenous participation in the military from 2001 to 2009 was an intricately woven story of precolonial Indigenous values, a history of racist Euro-American invasion, and the many material reasons for Native American enlistment, including benefits for families and communities. It is a story that begins in the emergence of Indigenous Peoples on the earth. It is greater than the boundaries, the weapons, the policies, and the suffering that are the roots and product of what has become the United States of America.

This research has raised many questions that beg for further research: Why do Indigenous families, communities, and nations have to sacrifice

Indigenous youth so that they can follow dreams of military service? How can Indigenous Peoples address the structures that prevent them from re-creating Indigenous institutions of warriorhood? How can we provide the means for our youth to protect Native homelands through our own terms? As Native nations, could Indigenous Peoples require the United States to honor our history, our treaties, and our sovereignty through ensuring that all Native recruits and veterans are provided exceptional career and educational counseling by Native leaders in the military? How can Indigenous Peoples make their own decisions of what constitutes a *just* war and what is really worth the lives of their children?

In considering the topic of Indigenous participation in the military in the context of health and wellness, the best way to understand the concept of Native American veterans' well-being is to view it through the narratives of those individuals who made the journey and returned with grace and knowledge. By considering the stories of Native veterans, we can best understand what it means to sacrifice lives for the greater good of society. It is not to sacrifice a life for American constructs of freedom but to sacrifice time, served in the military, to come out with a stronger appreciation of true Indigenous values and save the lives of future generations from the devastating symptoms of colonization.

REFERENCES

Brayboy, Bryan. 2005. "Toward a Tribal Critical Race Theory in Education." *Urban Review* 37, no. 5 (December): 425–46. https://doi.org/10.1007/s11256-005 -0018-y.

Brickman, Stephanie, Dennis M. McInerney, and Amy Martin. 2009. "Examining the Valuing of Schooling as a Motivational Indicator of American Indian Students: Perspectives Based on a Model of Future Oriented Motivation and Self-Regulation." *Journal of American Indian Education* 48, no. 2: 33–54. https://www.jstor.org/stable/24398744.

Bush, George W. 2001. Address to a Joint Session of Congress and the American People. https://georgewbush-whitehouse.archives.gov/news/releases/2001/09 /20010920-8.html.

CEHIP Incorporated, in partnership with Rodger Bucholz, William Fields, and Ursula P. Roach. 1996. *20th Century Warriors: Native American Participation in the United States Military*. Washington, D.C.: U.S. Department of Defense. https://www.history.navy.mil/research/library/online-reading-room/title-list -alphabetically/t/american-indians-us-military.html.

Cook-Lynn, Elizabeth. 2007. *New Indians, Old Wars*. Urbana: University of Illinois Press.

Fischer, Hannah, Kim Klarman, and Mari-Jana Oboroceanu. 2008. American War and Military Operations Causalities: Lists and Statistics. CRS Report RL32492. Washington, D.C.: Congressional Research Service, updated May 14, 2008. https://www.everycrsreport.com/files/20080514_RL32492_fbb25fcfa566a0b573 bfbcf1b84b144088bb205d.pdf.

Hartung, William D. 2021. "Profits of War: Corporate Beneficiaries of the Post-9/11 Pentagon Spending Surge." Watson Institute International & Public Affairs Brown University, September 13, 2021. https://watson.brown.edu/costs ofwar/files/cow/imce/papers/2021/Profits%20of%20War_Hartung_Costs%20 of%20War_Sept%2013%2C%202021.pdf.

Huyser, Kimberly R., Sofia Locklear, Connor Sheehan, Brenda L. Moore, and John S. Butler. 2021. "Consistent Honor, Persistent Disadvantage: American Indian and Alaska Native Veteran Health in the National Survey of Veterans." *Journal of Aging and Health* 33, no. S7–8: S68–81. https://doi.org/10.1177/0898 2643211014034.

Iraq Body Count. 2011. "Documented Civilian Deaths from Violence." https://www.iraqbodycount.org/.

Iraq Coalition Casualty Count. 2009. "Operation Iraqi Freedom and Operation Enduring Freedom Casualties." http://icasualties.org/.

Korshak, Lauren, Donna L. Washington, and Stephanie Birdwell. n.d. "Indian/Alaska Native Veterans Fact Sheet." U.S. Department of Veteran Affairs, Veterans Health Administration, Office of Health Equity. Accessed June 19, 2023. https://www.va.gov/HEALTHEQUITY/docs/American_Indian_Heritage _Month_Fact_Sheet.pdf.

Military Times. n.d. "Marine Lance Cp. Emilian D. Sanchez." Accessed July 28, 2023. https://thefallen.militarytimes.com/marine-lance-cpl-emilian-d-sanchez /2507783.

Miller, Raymond B., and Stephanie J. Brickman. 2004. "A Model of Future-Oriented Motivation and Self-Regulation." *Educational Psychology Review* 16, no. 1 (March): 9–33. http://dx.doi.org/10.1023/B:EDPR.0000012343 .96370.39.

National Center for Veterans Analysis and Statistics. 2017. "American Indian and Alaska Native Veterans: 2017." https://www.va.gov/vetdata/docs/Special Reports/AIAN.pdf.

National Museum of the United States Army. n.d. "Biographies: Lori Ann Piestewa." Accessed July 28, 2023. https://www.thenmusa.org/biographies/lori -ann-piestewa/.

Newcomb, Steven T. 2008. *Pagans in the Promised Land: Decoding the Doctrine of Christian Discovery*. New York: Fulcrum Pub.

O'Connor, Phillip, and Kevin Crowe. 2008. "Commitment to Military Strong in Menominee Tribe." *St. Louis Post-Dispatch*, May 17, 2008. https://thesouthern .com/news/commitment-to-military-strong-in-menominee-tribe/article_fc63 ffbf-0bd7-5811-8282-e0b0e9ca9778.html.

Pewewardy, Cornel. 2005. "Ideology, Power, and the Miseducation of Indigenous Peoples in the United States." In *For Indigenous Eyes Only: A Decolonization Handbook*, edited by Waziyatawin Angela Wilson and Michael Yellow Bird, 139–56. Santa Fe, NM: School of American Research.

PowWows.com. n.d. "What Is a Native American Pow Wow?" Accessed June 19, 2023. https://www.powwows.com/main/native-american-pow-wow/.

Sallah, Michael, and Mitch Weiss. 2006. *Tiger Force: A True Story of Men and War*. New York: Little, Brown.

Schwartz, Mainon A. 2023. *The 574 Federally Recognized Indian Tribes in the United States*. CRS Report R47414. Washington, D.C.: Congressional Research Service, February 8, 2023. https://crsreports.congress.gov/product/pdf /R/R47414.

Suina, Joseph. 2005. Lecture delivered at the Institute for American Indian Education, Albuquerque, NM, September, 2005.

Tsinnajinnie, Leola Roberta. 2011. "Examining the Indigenous Relationship Between Education and the United States Military from 2001–2009." PhD diss., University of New Mexico. https://digitalrepository.unm.edu/educ_llss_etds/45/.

Yellow Bird, Michael. 2006. "Why Are Indigenous Soldiers in Iraq?" *Arikara Consciousness* (blog). June 26, 2006. https://arikaraconsciousness.blogspot .com/2007/06/indigenous-professors-against-us-led.html.

Yellow Bird, Michael. 2012. "A BROWN Paper on the Iraq War and the Resurrection of Traditional Principals of Just War." In *For Indigenous Minds Only: A Decolonization Handbook*, edited by Waziyatawin Angela Wilson and Michael Yellow Bird, 157–78. Santa Fe, NM: School for Advanced Research Press.

LEGAL RESOURCES

American Indian Religious Freedom Act, Pub. L. No. 95–341, 92 Stat. 469 (1978)

Johnson v. M'Intosh, 21 U.S. 543 (1823)

No Child Left Behind Act, Pub. L. No. 107–110, 115 Stat. 1425 (2001)

PART II

COVID-19 IMPACTS

KAREN JARRATT-SNIDER AND
MARIANNE O. NIELSEN

S ARS-COV-2, THE VIRUS THAT causes what we now commonly call COVID-19, continues to have devastating effects on Indigenous communities worldwide. As we noted in the introduction, COVID-19 was the leading cause of death among American Indians and Alaska Natives in 2020 (HHS 2022). Immersed as we are in the tragedies that have overtaken Indigenous nations, communities, and individuals here in the United States, it is sometimes difficult to remember that, in some respects, for many Indigenous Peoples outside the country, things are significantly worse, so that they are "disproportionately affected by epidemics and other crises" (UN DESA 2020). Indigenous Peoples make up about 6 percent of the world's population (UN DESA 2020), and according to the United Nations Expert Mechanism on the Right of Indigenous Peoples (EMRIP 2020),

> Many indigenous peoples live in remote regions difficult to access and often inaccessible. Even prior to this crisis, they experienced higher rates of health risks, poorer health and greater unmet needs in respect to health care than their non-indigenous counterparts. Indigenous peoples were already disadvantaged in terms of access to quality health care and were more vulnerable to numerous health problems, in particular pandemics. The social determinants of health such as safe drinking water and a suffi-

cient, balanced diet . . . and sanitation were not fulfilled before the crisis. Moreover, the expropriation of indigenous lands and natural resources and the increase in conflicts in their territories were already placing indigenous peoples in a particularly precarious position.

UN DESA (n.d.) also points to the lack of essential preventative measures such as "clean water, soap, disinfectant, etc.," the lack of access to health-care services, and poorly equipped and understaffed local medical facilities. Unfortunately, many Indigenous Peoples in the United States suffer from these same dangerous conditions, including people from the Navajo Nation, which has one of the largest Native nation citizen populations and is home to the largest reservation in the United States. (Navajo Nation Wind, n.d.). Navajo Nation lands extend from Arizona into both Utah and New Mexico, making the geographic size of the nation's lands larger than that of several U.S. states (Navajo Nation Wind, n.d.). Much of the nation's lands are in rural areas, and many Navajo families are without running water at home. According to the Navajo Water Project (n.d.), Navajo people pay sixty-seven times more for water, which they must haul, than those who enjoy running water piped into homes. Water is precious and its scarcity forces families to choose between using it for various critical needs: to sustain livestock, to cook, to wash hands for COVID safety, or the many other vital functions of water in daily life. The Navajo Nation is not alone, in the United States or the world, in having to deal with issues that exacerbate the provision of health care to its citizens. Extractive industries in particular are to blame for adverse effects on Indigenous individuals' health in the United States and worldwide. Often, mining sites produce toxic water, air, and other unhealthy conditions impacting Indigenous people (Jarratt-Snider and Nielsen 2020).

EMRIP (2020) goes on to call on the states within which Indigenous Peoples live to "fulfill their human rights obligations, guided by the UN Declaration on the Rights of Indigenous Peoples, to protect the health and lives of indigenous people."

Many Indigenous nations are finding their own solutions when the state can't or won't. Their de facto sovereignty once again demonstrates the resilience of Indigenous Peoples as they use traditional knowledge and methods, such as sealing off their territories and ordering isolation to protect their population from threats like COVID (UN DESA, n.d.).

As the authors in this section point out, the ongoing health disparities that impact Indigenous communities in the United States contribute to multiplying the impacts of COVID. The lack of running water made sanitation difficult, living in multigenerational housing with inadequate space for isolation and quarantine made protecting elders nearly impossible, and the initial lack of protective personal equipment (PPE) meant there was no way to stop the virus's spread. In addition, isolated homes without electricity meant little access to vital media information and news. During the pandemic, health-care workers couldn't go home without risking infecting their families, so they had to live in trailers or motels. Here at Northern Arizona University (NAU), while we were using remote learning, we had Indigenous students sitting in parking lots to access Wi-Fi hot spots, uploading and downloading class materials. Some drove over three hundred miles to get access. While the nations were on lockdown, many students couldn't even do that and fell behind in their assignments. They persevered, though, even after losing family members or falling sick themselves. The Navajo Nation lost a K–12 teacher whom the authors personally knew through our work with the Institute for Native-serving Educators at NAU. As far as we know, we didn't lose any NAU Indigenous students or faculty to COVID, though some students are suffering from long COVID and grieving the loss of relatives (personal communications from students). Most Indigenous communities and families were not as fortunate.

In chapter 4, Begay, Petillo, and Goldtooth describe how the COVID pandemic provided an opportunity for nation rebuilding by the Navajo government. Native nation building, as the authors explain, is a formula for Indigenous self-determination. They point to the resilience of Indigenous nations and communities in identifying opportunities to overcome the many issues that have confronted Indigenous communities, in the United States and globally, over the years.

Haskie provides a case study in chapter 5 that describes how one small Diné community reacted to the communications issued by the Navajo Nation government about the use of PPE and other preventive measures as part of its response to the pandemic. The Navajo Nation took advantage of every media source available to it, including television, radio, newspapers, and social media, but due to the isolation and lack of electricity in many homes, and the lockdowns that prevented people from traveling, people could not access enough information fast enough. Along with chapter 4, Haskie's chapter points to the resilience of not only Indigenous individuals but whole communities.

The majority of the American population very likely gets its knowledge of Indian Country health issues not in school settings but from media sources such as newspapers, online streaming, television, and social media. Educational textbooks are certainly not doing the job of adequately teaching non-Indigenous and Indigenous students about the truth of colonization and its impacts on the health and well-being of Indigenous Peoples and individuals (see Loewen 1995). The representations of Indigenous Peoples, lifeways, and issues found in non-Indigenous media are biased toward the negative and are often stereotypical and bleak. As Kunze and Camarillo point out in chapter 6, however, there are Indigenous publications and news sources, whose numbers are growing all the time. An excellent example is *Indian Country Today*, an independent multimedia news outlet. Such media outlets are not well known outside of Indian Country, but they are worth finding for those who want to understand Indigenous issues from the perspectives of those most affected by them and want information about Indigenous solutions to these issues. By focusing on one recent and tragic health crisis, COVID-19, Kunze and Camarillo show how inadequately mainstream newspapers portrayed the pandemic's consequences in Indian Country. They point out how the resilience and adaptive abilities of Indigenous nations and communities are not seen as newsworthy, which perpetuates stereotypes and negative public perceptions of Indigenous Peoples. It would be very interesting to find out how news coverage in other countries contributes to negative perceptions of Indigenous Peoples and, very likely, the neglect of their human right to good health—not just during this latest pandemic but overall.

REFERENCES

EMRIP (United Nations Expert Mechanism on the Rights of Indigenous Peoples). 2020. "COVID Yet Another Challenge for Indigenous Peoples." April 6, 2020. https://www.un.org/develop ment/desa/indigenouspeoples/covid-19/statements-by-the-unpfii -and-un-mandated-bodies-to-address-indigenous-peoples-issues .html.

HHS (U.S. Department of Health and Human Services). 2022. *How Increased Funding Can Advance the Mission of the Indian Health Service to Improve Health Outcomes for American Indians/Alaska Natives.* Report No. HP-2022–21. Washington, D.C.: Office of the Assistant Secretary for Planning and Evaluation, July 2022. https://aspe .hhs.gov/reports/funding-ihs.

Jarratt-Snider, Karen, and Marianne O. Nielsen, eds. 2020. *Indigenous Environmental Justice.* Tucson: University of Arizona Press.

Loewen, James W. 1995. *Lies My Teacher Told Me: Everything Your American History Textbook Got Wrong.* New York: Simon & Schuster.

Navajo Nation Wind. n.d. "Navajo Nation Profile." Accessed June 20, 2023. https://navajoprofile.wind.enavajo.org/.

Navajo Water Project. n.d. "About the Project." Accessed March 4, 2022. https://www.navajowaterproject.org/project-specifics.

UN DESA (United Nations Department of Economic and Social Affairs). n.d. "COVID-19 and Indigenous Peoples." Accessed March 4, 2022. https://www.un.org/development/desa/indigenouspeoples /covid-19.html.

UN DESA (United Nations Department of Economic and Social Affairs). 2020. "Indigenous Peoples and the COVID-19 Pandemic: Considerations." Blog post. May 4, 2020. https://www.un.org/develop ment/desa/indigenouspeoples/covid-19/statements-by-the-unpfii -and-un-mandated-bodies-to-address-indigenous-peoples-issues .html.

4

INDIGENOUS NATION REBUILDING

Pandemic-Tested Sovereignty, Health, and Resilience

MANLEY A. BEGAY JR., APRIL D. J. PETILLO,
AND CAROL GOLDTOOTH

NORTH AMERICAN INDIGENOUS SOCIETIES have approached this century with shared goals of political sovereignty, social self-determination, and economic viability built from their self-governance powers. Since the mid-1970s, U.S. Indigenous nations and, more recently, Canadian First Nations have prioritized and revived these Indigenous self-governance goals into a resurgence of governing powers not previously seen. This focus means more Indigenous nations have defined their political, social, and economic hopes on their terms, assuming governance previously forcibly managed by outsiders. Thus, Indigenous nations and leaders currently address the daunting challenges that *all* nations face, with the added complicated maneuvering of often unwilling state systems.

These challenges, or "sovereignty tests," are not managed through a magical process. Indigenous nations have proven that systematic, measured decision-making led by specific community needs, priorities, and values ensures self-determined governance success, no matter the circumstances. General governance challenges include developing, maintaining, and sustaining governing institutions, culturally appropriate political systems, and viable economies. This Indigenous governance resurgence has amplified Indigenous nations' approaches to maintaining and preserving Indigenous languages and culture; effectively managing the environment and natural resources; negotiating complex relationships with the federal government, states, and other entities; improving health; and advancing education. Increasingly, Indigenous nations are using this newfound political context to redefine the terms of successful governance, rebuilding their nations on their terms—especially when relying on other systems that encourage powerlessness, such as global medical communities.

Indigenous nations' responses to the COVID-19 pandemic and its impacts offer insight into governmental "resilience in action," or Indigenous governments' capacity to recover, if not grow, from unexpected difficulties quickly. This chapter examines the responses of several nations but focuses specifically on the experience and responses of the Cherokee Nation located in Oklahoma as a story illuminating self-determined action to ensure the safety of its citizens and sovereignty in the face of a global pandemic.

In this chapter, we explore early lessons about Indigenous nation rebuilding in such crises through brief vignettes of how some across the vast and varied terrains and cultures of Indigenous nations fared during the pandemic. We highlight initial Indigenous concerns about the pandemic's early impact on Indigenous Country,[1] considering the early responses of the Lummi Nation of Washington State, Havasupai Tribe of Arizona, and Cowessess First Nation of Saskatchewan. The bulk of this chapter highlights the Cherokee Nation's response as a case study, within which we comprehensively analyze the Indigenous nation rebuilding potential presented by COVID-19. We conclude with the lessons Indigenous nations' responses illustrate about resilience in the face of a global crisis.

INDIGENOUS NATION REBUILDING IN A PUBLIC HEALTH POLICY CONTEXT

Many Indigenous nations are not simply building but resurrecting and adapting (or rebuilding) practices their communities have engaged in

---

1. What we discuss as Indigenous Country and Indigenous America covers both formally recognized Indigenous land as well as Indigenous claims ignored by the U.S. federal government, including the communities heavily influenced by and bordering this land. While U.S. and Canadian law may distinguish between legally defined Indigenous territory, these borders can be porous. Airborne viruses, as well as the people impacted by them, cross such legally defined borders with ease. Therefore, Indigenous governments' concerns and, in some cases, assertions of sovereignty necessarily cross these legal borders as well.

some form since time immemorial. Indigenous nation rebuilding details the approaches to governance and elements shared by Indigenous nations that have successfully managed and overcome contemporary community and economic development challenges on *their* terms. Grounded in nearly five decades of research by chapter co-author Dr. Manley Begay Jr., the Harvard Project on American Indian Economic Development (founded in 1987), the Native Nations Institute (founded in 2001), and the Tribal Leadership Initiative (founded in 2014), Indigenous nation rebuilding has two primary goals: to better understand sustained, successful Indigenous nation development and to amplify stories of hope concerning Indigenous governance and leadership. Research to this end has identified the following five critical elements of effective Indigenous development:

- willingness to assert sovereignty and governing power or authority in decision-making
- effective dispute resolution and institutional processes for a capable bureaucracy with minimal "politicking"
- insistence on cultural match or alignment such that community beliefs about what authority looks like and how it operates remain identifiable and visible in that nation's governance practices
- core commitment(s) to long-term, future-facing strategies that orient all actions toward building sustainable solutions
- leadership capable of purposely creating and sustaining fundamental changes *with* instead of *for* the community or without continued community involvement

This theoretical framework can sound like a community-grounded economic approach—and for some, nation building is purely economic. As sociologists and public policy scholars and practitioners, we firmly believe that healthy communities are a requirement of any sound, healthy, and sustainable economic development. These ideas also resonate when thinking about Indigenous community development, capacity building, and policymaking beyond economics. This resonance has been incredibly vibrant in how numerous Indigenous nations have wrestled with keeping their communities safe during a pandemic. From that broad approach to understanding Indigenous nation rebuilding, the authors consider the following components key to developing a successful response to the COVID-19 pandemic: 1) forward-thinking, purposive leadership unafraid to assert sovereignty and willing to "walk the walk" by providing clear direction paralleled with the nation's mission and vision; 2) following the science and using technology in a way that matches the Indigenous nation's mission and values; and 3) health-care investments that align with Indigenous nation needs and ideals.

THE IMPORTANCE OF SELF-DETERMINED PANDEMIC RESPONSES IN INDIGENOUS COUNTRY

THE LUMMI NATION OF WASHINGTON STATE DID NOT WAIT ON OTHERS TO SAVE THEM

Indigenous nations across the United States watched non-Indigenous governmental responses to the pandemic seemingly as a cautionary tale. Where some states and metropolitan areas lagged, several Indigenous governments quickly responded with extensive mitigation and prevention measures that included infrastructural adjustments, community-minded policies, and public health services for those who contracted COVID-19 and those who were concerned about contracting it. One example of this decisive approach is the Pacific Northwest Lummi Nation. In March 2020, four months after news broke of a novel, deadly virus endangering China's population, the Lummi prepared to open a field hospital to treat those who had become ill with the coronavirus. The field hospital was part of more extensive mitigation and prevention measures the nation believed necessary to curb the coronavirus's expected health impacts. As rising coronavirus cases and accompanying health issues seemingly blindsided the Seattle, Washington, area, the Lummi Tribal Council declared a state of emergency and planned their response. The nation, a sovereign entity with all its accompanying powers and authority, set these efforts into motion grounded in a steadfast self-determining spirit. Dr. Dakotah Lane, the executive medical director of the Lummi Tribal Health Center, explained, "The Lummi believe in controlling our own destiny. We don't count on help reaching us, but the hospital is something we can do to help the community" (Lakhani 2020).

The Lummi's bold sense of autonomy, independence, and self-governance informed their COVID-19 pandemic efforts. Early in the pandemic, governmental decisions were made to close the casino and execute established emergency health response codes (Hiraldo, James, and Carroll 2021). The Lummi Nation is not the only Indigenous nation to assert its sovereignty by manifesting bold governmental actions while protecting its citizenry during the COVID-19 pandemic—and such trailblazing nations will not be the last. The reason for that is simple: questions arising from these efforts, and other related questions, directly concern the well-being and future of Indigenous nations, their governments, and their people. Political scientists have long discussed how nations learn to assert themselves by following the examples of other nations that have done so successfully. Indigenous nations are no different, building success by exploring and adapting models set by other Indigenous nations. Historical moments such as this worldwide pandemic call to these discussions Indigenous leaders, federal authorities, and policymakers hoping to build effective and efficient governing systems.

THE COWESSESS FIRST NATION OF SASKATCHEWAN RESPONDS WITH PURPOSE-DRIVEN LEADERSHIP

Indigenous nations also employed effective governance practices to address COVID-19 concerns at a time when non-Indigenous nations resorted to political infighting and/or "not it" games across levels of government. Where individual city, county, state, and provincial officials struggled to coordinate with public health entities to protect and inform the public, several Indigenous governments exemplified what we call purpose-driven leadership.

Purpose-driven leadership is "when a leader prioritizes their purpose and values over anything else when making decisions on behalf of the [organization]" (Herrington 2021). Purposive leadership focuses on a collective future, ensuring continuance across multiple generations. This kind of leadership operates with a goal beyond prosperity, using a collective rights–oriented spirit and collaborative approach as the standard for measuring "a good future." The Cowessess First Nation of Saskatchewan exemplified such leadership during the pandemic.

Cowessess First Nation leaders began preparing for the novel coronavirus in February 2020. As the pandemic emerged, the nation immediately established its COVID-19 task force of council members and directors. By the second week of March 2020, preparations turned into implementation with the launch of the nation's Emergency Management and Communicable Disease Plans and Flagging System (Cowessess First Nation 2021; Cadmus Delorme, interview with Manley A. Begay Jr., June 15, 2022). Chief Cadmus Delorme acknowledges that teamwork among tribal leaders and directors, commitment to protecting on-reserve and off-reserve citizens, partnerships with neighboring grocery stores and companies, exercising jurisdiction, leadership foresight, and good communication systems were keys to alleviating the pandemic's impact (interview with Manley A. Begay Jr., June 15, 2022). These highly coordinated efforts seem to have been effective—the Cowessess First Nation's initial COVID-19 case was not recorded until January 2021, one year after the U.S. Centers for Disease Control and Prevention (CDC) sent a team to Washington State concerning the first reported case of the novel coronavirus (CDC 2023).

The Cowessess First Nation is remote, located about ninety miles east of what is now known as Regina in Canada's Saskatchewan province. Its geography forces the nation to rely on its own resources and ingenuity if challenges arise, and this did not change with the realization that the world was in the midst of a global pandemic. Given the pandemic confinement measures in effect, there needed to be communication mechanisms to ensure the Cowessess people's needs were being met. The nation's leaders were not new to exercising sovereignty and making their own decisions regarding the welfare and well-being of their citizens. As canceled public events and shutdowns loomed large, the Cowessess Nation quickly moved to technological solutions to ease pandemic-related communication burdens. Zoom meetings, social media (i.e., Facebook, YouTube, etc.), cellular systems, and other technology were the nation's mainstays for keeping its government on course. The task force initiated the nation's peacekeepers as communicators between its citizens and various governmental units to help respond to its people's needs.

This self-determined attitude encouraged the nation's fortuitous partnering with Lumeca to launch a pilot program for their virtual Health Pod, a first for North America before the pandemic. The Health Pod is "equipped with cameras, microphones, and a touchscreen and allows patients to access physician care virtually within minutes" (RedMane Technology 2020). In anticipation of the pandemic's outbreak, Chief Delorme stated that when the pandemic arrives at Cowessess in full force, "this pod will enhance the timeliness of service delivery. Also, in a time of COVID-19, reducing the risk means remaining at home as much as possible. Being able to talk privately with a specialist while staying home is a benefit to minimizing the risk" (interview with Manley A. Begay Jr., June 15, 2022). In addition to the virtual pod, Cowessess deliberately partnered with and implemented RedMane's mCase platform, which "easily supports any case management program, including those involving intake, assessment, eligibility, service planning, financial processing, and/or ongoing service delivery. It works in the office and in the field, even without Internet or cellular connectivity" (RedMane Technology 2020). This innovative case management system allowed Cowessess to track and monitor all who entered and left the community, thereby aiding in preventing the spread of the coronavirus. As Chief Delorme explained, "One of the challenges First Nations face is having access to our own data. With this technology, our COVID-19 task force was better able to make decisions based on understanding the patterns of behavior of our people during the pandemic" (interview with Manley A. Begay Jr., June 15, 2022).

THE HAVASUPAI TRIBE OF ARIZONA
PUT THE PEOPLE FIRST

At the height of the pandemic, the Havasupai Tribal Council exercised its sovereign authority, enacting Resolution 10–20, which temporarily closed one of the world's scenic wonders because of the threat of COVID-19. The Havasupai Tribe live at the bottom of the Grand Canyon, accessible only by an eight-mile trek on foot, by horseback, by helicopter, or by boat on the Colorado River. The temporary closure was extended by council resolution at least four times, with the last in effect through the end of 2022. "The health and safety of the many tourists who visit as well as our Tribal Members, employees, and consultants are very important to us," said Chairwoman Eva Kissoon. "The Tribal Council considered many options and determined that temporarily closing Supai to tourists at this time was the best decision" (Havasupai Tribal Council 2020). In addition to closing Supai, the council made the decision to quickly develop an emergency team and engage with an epidemiologist to assist the tribe in determining how to best protect the people.

While the Havasupai Tribe's economy depends heavily on tourism, the nation took its responsibility to its citizens seriously enough that it continued to halt tourist income long after many non-Indigenous nations gave in to economic pressures. Over forty-thousand tourists come annually to Supai's exquisite blue-green waterfalls and pristine landscapes. Nevertheless, Havasupai leadership was determined to proactively protect its people from the impact of the novel coronavirus. Tribal chairman Thomas Siyuja Sr. stated, "There are still so many unknowns with the new COVID-19 variants that for the health and safety of our tribal community, it is in the best interest to remain closed to tourists" (Silversmith 2022). Refusing to succumb to economic pressures paid off. Though some of the statistical data about COVID-19 among the Havasupai people is unavailable to the general public, what is available indicates no reported coronavirus cases through June 2021, unlike in the rest of the United States. The lack of new infections had the potential to prevent additional extensive public health costs and potentially devastating loss of Havasupai citizens. Additionally, we understand the Havasupai's choice to control information about their pandemic rates as an effort to prevent racial stereotyping and an assertion of their public health and data sovereignty, per the Indigenous collective and individual data rights outlined in the United Nations Declaration on the Rights of Indigenous Peoples (UNDRIP) (UNGA 2007).[2]

These three snapshots only highlight Indigenous-specific coronavirus concerns and responses. While each nation responded according to their unique Indigenous concerns, values, and traditional principles, they also all shared a self-determined focus on protecting their current citizens and futures. This shared focus is not a fluke; rather, it is a part of a process of persistent survival grounded in a history of outside interference in individual Indigenous nations' public health, economics, law, and society. The story of the Cherokee Nation's pandemic response illustrates

---

2. Generally, data sovereignty recognizes that data is subject to the laws and regulations of the geographic location where it is collected and processed. The goal is to protect sensitive, private data and ensure the data owner's control of its use. In an Indigenous context, the conversation about data is in relation to postcolonial state attempts to control Indigenous data and considers power differentials as well as historical contexts (GIDA 2019; UNGA 2007).

how these structural interferences require Indigenous self-determined resilience.

A PANDEMIC RESPONSE INFORMED BY NATION REBUILDING: THE CHEROKEE NATION CASE STUDY

A HISTORY AND PRESENT GROUNDED IN SURVIVANCE

Gerald Vizenor, a Minnesota Chippewa Tribe White Earth Reservation citizen, writer, and theorist, has used the idea of "survivance" to discuss Indigenous survival as a decidedly active and continual process instead of an end goal. Survivance recognizes that Indigenous Peoples continue to change in a distinctively resistant way. Vizenor anchors survivance as honoring cultural and traditional specificity within individual communities' adaptive social strategies. Survivance is more than existing as living historical tribal stereotypes; instead, it actively refashions those inherited cultures as evolving sources of strength (Vizenor 1999). Cherokee Nation history well illustrates survivance.

Creating opportunities from brushes with potential devastation is a long-cultivated skill of the Cherokee. Originally from what is now known as the southeastern United States, the Cherokee Nation's first European contact, through Hernando de Soto in 1540, began their trade and inter-relationships with other Europeans. Though eighteenth- and nineteenth-century treaties between the Cherokee and the British, including the 1835 Treaty of New Echota, inevitably increased European influence on the Cherokee economy, the Cherokee adapted and thrived: they created a fully functioning constitutional government, a flourishing economy, and a political identity, evidenced by Sequoyah's creation of the written Cherokee language and, eventually, the *Cherokee Phoenix*, a newspaper published in both Cherokee and English (Cherokee Nation 2023c).

Within two years of the *Cherokee Phoenix*'s inaugural year, the federal government precipitated unwarranted changes to U.S.-Indigenous relations, culminating in the 1830 Indian Removal Act. This act, and the Treaty of New Echota, forced many Cherokee to relocate to western lands—Oklahoma "Indian Territory." About sixteen thousand Cherokee were forced to journey to newly designated Indian Territory, and some four thousand Cherokee perished on the way (Cherokee Nation 2023c). Despite the challenges thrust upon the forcibly relocated, the Cherokee began nation rebuilding by ratifying a new constitution, establishing a new supreme court, and reviving vital Cherokee entities such as the newspaper, schools, businesses, and other forms of infrastructure. The Civil War interrupted Cherokee Nation rebuilding efforts in Indian Territory, dividing the Cherokee Nation and the United States. The Union's victory saw the Cherokee signing their last treaty with the United States in 1866 (Cherokee Nation 2023c).

After the Civil War ended, the Cherokee returned to Cherokee Nation rebuilding, only to have the push for Oklahoma statehood upend this process. Legislative interference, such as the Dawes Act of 1887 and the Curtis Act of 1898, paved the path to Oklahoma statehood. Amid white settler encroachment and the subsequent push to join lands of the "Five Civilized Tribes" with Oklahoma Territory, the Dawes Act was broad, sweeping legislation to regulate U.S. tribal territory land rights through severalty, which emphasized the individual instead of tribal/communal land rights and access and opened Indigenous lands for non-Indigenous occupation and westward expansion. The Curtis Act dissolved Indian Territory governments "by abolishing tribal courts and subjecting all persons in the territory to federal law" (Tatro, n.d.). Legislatively imposed U.S. schools, citizenship requirements, and political practices undermined Cherokee (and other among the five tribes) governance broadly, effectively dissolving the Cherokee Nation's infrastructure while making way for Oklahoma statehood a year later. These changes devastated the Cherokee, plaguing them with considerable poverty until the 1970s (Cherokee Nation 2023c).

The 1960s and 1970s civil rights, American Indian, Red Power, and Indian Self-Determination and Education Assistance Act movements paved the way for the Cherokee Nation to take back their governance and popularly elect Cherokee officials. Through the Principal Chiefs Act of 1970, the Cherokee Nation held its first election in nearly seventy years and ratified a new constitution. With this policy action grounded in the spirit of self-determination and new social movements, the Cherokee Nation once again renewed its rebuilding efforts (Cherokee Nation 2023c).

Today the Cherokee Nation is the second-largest Indigenous nation in the United States, after the Navajo Nation. The Cherokee Nation boasts over 390,000 citizens worldwide and more than 141,000 citizens residing within its northeastern Oklahoma boundaries. The Cherokee's self-determined policies have expanded through survivance as well. Partially based on the 1835 Treaty of New Echota's guarantee of the right to self-government under federal supervision, the Cherokee Nation claimed its sovereign right to prosecute offenses (instead of the United States) committed in the nation involving Native Americans in the landmark *McGirt v. Oklahoma* (2020). Though this case involves the Muscogee (Creek) Nation directly, the decision affirms the Cherokee, Chickasaw, Choctaw, Quapaw, and Seminole Nations' rights. This right stands despite the state's thirty-plus petitions to overrule the decision in the subsequent two years. The nation also provides its citizenry health and human services, education, employment, housing, economic and infrastructure development, environmental protection, and more. The Cherokee Nation and its subsidiaries are among the largest employers in northeastern Oklahoma, with approximately eleven thousand employees. Cherokee survivance has also shifted the economic relationships established for the nation in the eighteenth and nineteenth centuries. The Cherokee Nation had a more than $2.16 billion impact on the Oklahoma economy in 2018, before the initial brunt of the pandemic (Cherokee Nation 2023a).

THE LINK BETWEEN LANGUAGE AND CULTURE

The website of the Cherokee Nation (2023d) states, "The Cherokee Nation is committed to protecting our inherent sovereignty, preserving and promoting Cherokee culture, language, and values, and improving the quality of life for the next seven generations of Cherokee Nation citizens." This purposive mission underscores the link between language and culture with leadership and government among the Cherokee.

Linguists describe the Cherokee language as Iroquoian and polysynthetic. The primary U.S. government language training institution, the Foreign Service Institute, ranks Cherokee among the hardest for native English speakers to learn due to inherent linguistic and cultural differences. Today Cherokee is spoken fluently by an estimated two thousand people. Instead of an alphabet, written Cherokee uses a syllabary of eighty-five distinct characters representing the full spectrum of sounds used to speak the language. Cherokee traditional knowledge and language fluency have progressively declined, with the language now classified as endangered. Cherokee leaders issued a state of emergency in 2019, which led the nation to develop immersion schools and other similar measures to preserve and maintain the Cherokee language (Cherokee Nation 2023e). Deputy Principal Chief Bryan Warner, who also believes that knowing the language is an integral part of being Cherokee, said, "The Cherokee language, I believe, is the soul of the Cherokee people" (Cherokee One Feather 2019).

PANDEMIC IMPACTS ON CHEROKEE LANGUAGE AND CULTURE

Beyond policy, understanding the language decline seems uppermost in the minds of Cherokee leadership, a concern that only increased with the pandemic. Chuck Hoskin Jr., who was elected principal chief in 2019, connected Cherokee language concerns to the nation's vaccine rollout, since "Saving the language is in [Cherokee] national interest" (Brown 2021). This assessment is reasonable: the Cherokee have an estimated two thousand remaining speakers—many of whom are elders, considered one of the age groups most vulnerable to coronavirus-related mortality. Elders are held in high esteem in Indigenous societies because, as Principal Chief Hoskin explained, they are often "older members [of the society] who pass on cultural knowledge, oral histories, and traditional practices" (Brown 2021). Any elder loss reduces the number of Cherokee language speakers *and* access to people who operate as "libraries of lifeways, culture, stories, and language" for the community (Brown 2021). The Cherokee Nation has lost more than fifty fluent language speakers during the pandemic at the time of this writing—a shift reverberating across the nation with implications for several generations.

INDIGENOUS SPECIFIC VACCINATION CHALLENGES

Historically, vaccination and efficacy assessment in the United States and Canada has roots in the late eighteenth-century response to the impacts of infectious disease on significant world events such as large-scale wars (Smith, Wood, and Darden 2011). Many among the general public expressed concerns and even shock that COVID-19 vaccination is a "lightning rod" issue. However, vaccination has divided people along political lines since the international medical community began trying to address smallpox. Throughout this long social and political history, race, ethnicity, class, gender, and sexual identity have often negatively influenced the development, use, and accompanying vaccine-related surveillance—especially among minoritized populations. Thus, U.S. Indigenous health-care and vaccination is a complicated political enterprise.

The United States' current Indigenous health-care system blends the Indian Health Service (IHS) and tribally operated and urban Indian health-care hospitals and clinics. COVID-19 vaccine distribution efforts differ across states and Indigenous nations, sometimes impeded by community members' vaccine hesitancy. Among many reasons for this reluctance are mistrust of federal and state governments, concerns about vaccine safety, access problems such as site distance and transportation, and general politically fueled misinformation (Cordova 2022; Sanchez and Foxworth 2021). Further, Indigenous Peoples' hesitancy to trust U.S. government–distributed health mandates is not unwarranted; one need only consider that the IHS forced sterilization on American Indian women in the 1960s and 1970s. According to 1974 study by Dr. Connie Pinkerton-Uri, a Choctaw/Cherokee physician, the "Indian Health Service appeared to have 'singled out full-blooded Indian women for sterilization procedures'" (Kennedy 2019). Pinkerton-Uri's study also found that at least one in four American Indian women between the ages of fifteen and forty-four had been sterilized without consent (Kennedy 2019). These health-related injustices have informed the level of community trust for decades, and they will continue to create caution for generations to come—even when facing a public health concern such as the COVID-19 pandemic.

The U.S. Food and Drug Administration approved the Pfizer-BioNTech and Moderna COVID-19 vaccines in early December 2020—nine months after the first novel coronavirus reports from China. During that wait, the world debated and worried broadly about safety, access, and cost. People in minoritized and marginalized communities also weighed the dangers of vaccination in their particular contexts, considering their communal histories of inequity and injustice within medical practices, generally, and vaccination processes specifically. These concerns collided with governmental precautions about vaccine supply, distributed in the form of a four-phase vaccination rollout. The vaccination phases detailed in figure 4.1 determined the qualifying eligibility for and timing of access to preventative medicine, which could be the deciding variable between life and death.

For this case study, it is important to pay attention to the details of who was eligible for the vaccine in phase 1 of the process, per CDC guidelines (Kates, Tolbert, and Michaud 2021):

- Phase 1a—Health-care personnel and residents of long-term care facilities
- Phase 1b—Frontline essential workers and people aged 75 years and older
- Phase 1c—People aged 65–74 years and 16–64 years with underlying medical conditions

Other workers not mentioned are people in transportation and logistics, food service, housing construction and finance, information technology, communications, energy, law, media, public safety, and public health (see also Crawford 2021).

The Cherokee Nation received its first Pfizer-BioNTech vaccine shipment on December 14, 2020. Given Indigenous Peoples' previous challenging vaccination experiences and the COVID-19 vaccination process recommended by the CDC, Principal Chief Hoskin faced a significant decision amplified by Indigenous histories. How could he best manage vaccine distribution with the Cherokee Nation's particular needs, concerns, and priorities in mind?

DEVELOPING A CHEROKEE-SPECIFIC COVID-19 VACCINE ROLLOUT

Given the prospect that some Cherokee might hesitate around COVID-19 vaccination, the principal chief and his staff took several steps to build assurance that the vaccine was safe and beneficial. They did the following:

- tailored Cherokee Nation public health vaccine messaging to build trust
- asserted sovereignty and purpose-driven leadership decisions on vaccination priority

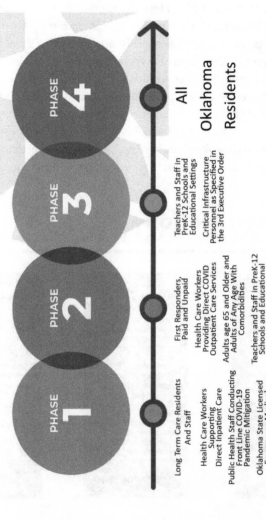

FIGURE 4.1 Oklahoma COVID-19 Vaccine Phases. Oklahoma State Department of Health, reprinted by the Oklahoma Bar Association.

- developed a health system and process owned by its people
- made significant investments in health care
- prioritized work to access the vaccine supply

Further, Principal Chief Hoskin's purposeful commitment to the Cherokee Nation mission of "preserving and promoting Cherokee culture, language, and values" (Cherokee Nation 2023d) put fluent Cherokee language speakers at the front of the conceptual vaccination line. Principal Chief Hoskin referred to this decision as the "biggest confidence builder" in the Cherokees' overall acceptance of the vaccine (Kaur 2021). Cherokee language speakers are highly respected and admired, and acknowledging this through the nation's vaccine policy brought vaccine acceptance into alignment with Cherokee Nation goals. "That's done something to create a sense of optimism among our people and also to boost the confidence

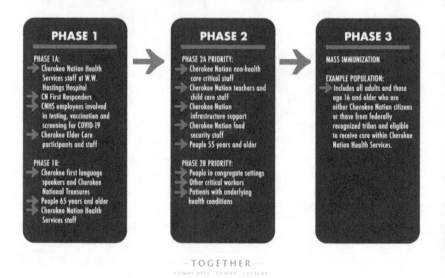

FIGURE 4.2 Cherokee Nation COVID-19 Vaccine Distribution Plan. (Cherokee Nation 2021a; see also Cherokee Nation 2021b)

of other Cherokees who see these very revered Cherokee elders, in many cases who are fluent speakers, getting the vaccines and celebrating it," stated Principal Chief Hoskin (Kaur 2021).

In early March 2021, the Cherokee Nation announced that it would make COVID-19 vaccines available to individuals who live within their nation's boundaries, including non-Natives (Cherokee Nation 2023b). According to Principal Chief Hoskin, this also stems from the Cherokee's understanding of how one functions as a part of community, family, and culture, and extends into public policy: "The Cherokee Nation is a good partner in our communities, and by working together, we can combat this deadly virus within our reservation and make more families safe. We're proud the Cherokee Nation can offer this service and give our communities the opportunity to be protected from COVID-19" (Polanksy 2021).

BUILDING FROM A PANDEMIC RESPONSE

The legacy of Cherokee investment in self-determined health-care continues. Bill John Baker, who served as principal chief from 2011 to 2019, has linked a survivance approach to Cherokee education with Cherokee public health investments. Principal Chief Baker explained, "Just as our ancestors grew their own teachers 150 years ago, we want to grow our own doctors" (McFarling 2020). In August 2020, the Cherokee Nation began erecting a medical school building, creating the United States' first tribally affiliated medical school, in a partnership with the Oklahoma State University College of Osteopathic Medicine. More than 20 percent of students in the inaugural class starting that fall identified as Native American. It is an unmistakably bold move to build a tribally affiliated medical school at this time but also unmistakably a hallmark of survivance.

KEYS TO PANDEMIC RESILIENCE AND SUCCESS

As Dr. Ashish Jha, dean of the Brown University School of Public Health, asserted, if the U.S. had responded the way the Cherokee Nation did, "we would be doing so much better . . . with tens of thousands of fewer deaths and probably a much more robust economy" (McFarling 2020).

Even amid a global pandemic, a look at localized public policy successes offers insight into creative problem-solving that can inspire hope in other similarly situated communities while amplifying self-determined policy and purpose-driven leadership decision-making that saves lives. The concerns highlighted earlier in this chapter framed Indigenous Country pandemic concerns distinctively connected to the realities of Indigenous life. We also discussed the following as Indigenous nation rebuilding–informed keys to a successful COVID pandemic response: 1) forward-thinking and purposive leadership unafraid to assert sovereignty and willing to "walk the walk," with the express purpose of fulfilling the mission and vision of the nation; 2) following the science in a way that matches the Indigenous nation's mission and values; and 3) health-care investments that align with Indigenous nation needs and ideals.

This Cherokee Nation vaccine rollout case study highlights where some of those concerns inform *better, more effective* policy originating in that distinctiveness and offers four key lessons for the future.

LESSON 1: CULTURALLY SPECIFIC PUBLIC POLICY MATTERS BROADLY

Indigenous sovereign rights cannot be overstated in the United States. The country's interlocking legal, political, social, and cultural history (and current reality) reminds us that we must foreground this conversation frequently. This reminder is especially salient considering the fact that most public policy touches Indigenous lives, recognizing that tribal sovereign rights should be a regular part of any public policy discussion. The National Indian Health Board chief executive officer, Stacey A. Bohlen, explains this connection in the context of the pandemic: "Tribes are sovereign nations with the autonomy to determine how to provide for the health care needs of their communities. For those that operate their own health systems, that meant being able to decide who should get priority for the vaccine. That autonomy allows tribes to adequately respond to the unique challenges they face" (Kaur 2021). Bohlen's points are particularly astute for the conversation about COVID-19 vaccine measures and processes but can be broadly applied.

Principal Chief Hoskin consistently embodied a lack of fear in asserting Cherokee sovereignty. He led conversations about the Cherokee Nation pandemic response and vaccine distribution, foregrounding the nation's sovereign rights and, ultimately, policymaking informed by community perspectives, values, and mission. This self-determined, community-defined approach to thinking through and acting on the health-care needs of the Cherokee also informs the nation's continued pandemic response, including initiating the tribally affiliated medical school in collaboration with the Oklahoma State University College of Osteopathic Medicine. As noted in the quote beginning this section of the chapter, such leadership lessons can, and do, have much broader impacts.

LESSON 2: PRIORITIZING COMMUNITY PERSPECTIVES MATTERS

This case study also shows that Indigenous policy that prioritizes community cultural perspectives addresses public health concerns more powerfully. This kind of prioritizing is beneficial even if it does not neatly align with global dictates. This prioritizing also follows the scientific research on public health efficacy and the science on mitigating COVID-19's spread across communities. Dr. Ashish Jha explains that the Cherokee Nation's vaccine-related culturally informed choices illustrate sound policymaking practices: "The tribe's COVID response meets the approval of global health leaders. It's very impressive. It's a reminder of how much leadership matters and how even under difficult circumstances, with limited resources, you can make a huge difference. It fits with what I've seen in the world. You see countries like Vietnam. They're not a wealthy country, but they've been following the science and doing a great job" (McFarling 2020). And in this instance, alignment with the Cherokee Nation's mission and values proved essential to meeting overall vaccination goals.

LESSON 3: HEALTH-CARE INVESTMENTS MATTER

In general, the United States "is a country that doesn't make access to health care just part of being a citizen. Because of that, there's uneven access to health care across the country. That's a problem during good times, and 'it's certainly a problem during the pandemic,'" says Principal Chief Hoskin (Kaur 2021). The disparities stratified across the United

States, especially in the early days of the pandemic, seem to support this sentiment. The Cherokee Nation sought a different health-care experience for its citizenry—one that better aligned with Cherokee needs and ideals. The nation spent the past decade shoring up its health-care system, which is now the most extensive tribally operated health system in the United States. That decision and the resulting robust infrastructure allowed the nation to set up a call center early and reach eligible citizens efficiently. Such efficiencies are essential to reducing loss of life during all pandemic stages, for the general public and for those providing lifesaving services. Michele Marshall, a nurse manager who oversees nursing staff at the new Cherokee Nation Health Services, underscores that point: "The facility is breathtaking to look at, and when you get into the logistics, it's mind-blowing. We have separate clinics with air exchange and negative air pressure. My staff feels very safe" (McFarling 2020). Now, as the additional impacts of the COVID-19 pandemic reverberate into high burnout rates among medical staff and over one million lives lost across the United States, we can learn from the Cherokee Nation's successes. Principal Chief Hoskin shared this powerful lesson for all nations, Indigenous or not: "You've got to invest in health care during the good times. Make it a priority for your nation and make it universally accessible for your citizens" (Kaur 2021).

LESSON 4: PURPOSE-DRIVEN LEADERSHIP MATTERS

The three lessons outlined above would be impossible without people committed to purposeful leadership grounded in tribally specific principles and values. Cherokee Nation leadership made choices to engage U.S. public policy in a way that prioritized Cherokee values and its overall mission, and thus effectively continued to discourage Cherokee vaccine reluctance. These efforts highlight that community perspectives and values are essential to any successful coronavirus-related public policy used in the United States. Further, rather than rest after successful vaccine implementation, Cherokee Nation leadership focused on the future by investing in its health-care infrastructure in ways that may ensure greater preparedness for future pandemics. These actions are hallmarks of outstanding leadership. Additionally, the consistent, committed focus on tribally specific solutions grounded in self-determined agency connecting these actions elevates them within an Indigenous nation rebuilding framework.

REFERENCES

Brennan, Natasha. 2022. "Lummi Nation Chairman Talks Culture, Language and Leading the Tribe Through COVID." *News Tribune*, May 27, 2022. https://www.thenewtribune.com/news/state/washington/article254869612.html.

Brown, Alex. 2021. "Racing to Save Languages and Cultures, Native American Tribes Rapidly Roll Out Vaccines." *In These Times*, February 18, 2021. https://inthesetimes.com/article/native-american-covid-vaccine-rollout.

CDC Mueum (David J. Sencer CDC Museum). 2023. "COVID-19 Timeline." Last updated March 15, 2023. https://www.cdc.gov/museum/timeline/covid 19.html.

Cherokee Nation. 2021a. "Cherokee Nation COVID-19 Vaccination Distribution Plan." February 3, 2021. https://health.cherokee.org/media/0cxpofht/vaccine -rollout-plan-february-2021-3.pdf.

Cherokee Nation. 2021b. "Cherokee Nation Moves to Phase 2B of COVID-19 Vaccination Plan." News release, February 10, 2021. https://anadisgoi.com /index.php/government-stories/501-cherokee-nation-moves-to-phase-2b-of -covid-19-vaccination-plan.

Cherokee Nation. 2023a. "About the Nation." Last updated February 9, 2023. https://www.cherokee.org/about-the-nation/.

Cherokee Nation. 2023b. "Health Services." Last updated January 10, 2023. https://health.cherokee.org/.

Cherokee Nation. 2023c. "History." Last updated June 9, 2023. https://www.cherokee.org/about-the-nation/history/.

Cherokee Nation 2023d. "Home." Last updated April 27, 2023. https://www.cherokee.org/.

Cherokee Nation. 2023e. "Language Department." Last updated June 21, 2023. https://language.cherokee.org.

Cherokee One Feather. 2019. "Cherokee Nation Chief Announces Largest Language Initiative in Tribe's History." September 29, 2019. https://theonefeather.com/2019/09/29/cherokee-nation-chief-announces-largest-language-initia tive-in-tribes.

Cherokee Phoenix. 2021. "Cherokee Nation Enters Phase 2A of COVID-19 Vaccine Distribution Plan." January 20, 2021. https://www.cherokeephoenix.org /health/cherokee-nation-enters-phase-2a-of-covid-19-vaccine-distribution -plan/article_e1741e22-4a47-565c-b930-adf964a7e8b2.html.

Cordova, Gilbert. 2022. "Why COVID-19 Vaccine Hesitancy Persists Among Native Americans." *ABC10 News*, January 26, 2022. https://www.abc10.com /article/news/community/race-and-culture/covid-19-vaccine-hesitancy-native -american-population/103-7545408f-29de-41c2-a74a-7832b50e0464.

Cowessess First Nation. 2021. *Annual Report, 2019–2020*. Cowessess, SK: Cowessess Ventures Ltd. https://issuu.com/cowessessfn/docs/cfn_2020_annual_report_.

Crawford, Grant D. 2021. "COVID Vaccination Phases Detailed for Cherokee Nation, Other Residents of Tribe's Capital." *Talequah Daily Press*, January 5, 2021. https://www.tahlequahdailypress.com/news/covid-vaccination-phases -detailed-for-cherokee-nation-other-residents-of-tribes-capital/article_fecc 6b53-9bf7-5426-acb0-ff5653f76b99.html.

Dungan, Ron. 2021. "How Arizona's Havasupai Tribe Has Kept COVID-19 Out of Its Community." *Cronkite News*, April 5, 2021. https://cronkitenews.azpbs .org/2021/04/05/how-arizonas-havasupai-tribe-has-resisted-covid-19/.

GIDA (Global Indigenous Data Alliance). n.d. "CARE Principles for Indigenous Data Governance." Accessed June 26, 2023. https://www.gida-global.org/care.

Havasupai Tribal Council. 2020. "The Havasupai Tribal Council to Suspend Tourism for 30 Days in Response to COVID-19 Pandemic." *Indian Country Today*, March 16, 2020. https://indiancountrytoday.com/the-press-pool/the -havasupai-tribal-council-to-suspend-tourism-for-30-days-in-response-to -covid-19-pandemic.

Herrington, Emily. 2021. "What Is Purpose-Driven Leadership?" Sidecar blog. March 5, 2021. https://www.sidecarglobal.com/organizational-culture/what-is -purpose-driven-leadership/#:~:text=Purpose%2Ddriven%20leadership%20is %20when.

Hiraldo, Danielle, Kyra James, and Stephanie Russo Carroll. 2021. "Case Report: Indigenous Sovereignty in a Pandemic: Tribal Codes in the United States as Preparedness." *Frontiers in Sociology* 6: article 617995 (March). https://doi.org /10.3389/fsoc.2021.617995.

Hunter, Chad. 2020. "Cherokee Nation Receives First Batch of COVID-19 Vaccine." *Cherokee Phoenix*, December 15, 2020. https://www.cherokeephoenix .org/health/cherokee-nation-receives-first-batch-of-covid-19-vaccine/article _0207b875-8c41-5b6e-a396-885c79c7fc48.html.

Indian Country Today. 2020. "Lumeca Partners with Cowessess First Nation to Connect Physicians and Patients by Launching Canada's First Virtual Healthcare Pod." July 21, 2020. https://indiancountrytoday.com/the-press -pool/lumeca-partners-with-cowessess-first-nation-to-connect-physicians-and -patients-by-launching-canadas-first-virtual-healthcare-pod.

Indian Country Today. 2021. "Havasupai Tribal Council Extends Tourism Suspension Until February 2022: Decision Made Due to Ongoing Impact of COVID-19." June 14, 2021. https://indiancountrytoday.com/the-press-pool/havasupai-tribal-council-extends-tourism-suspension-until-february-2022.

Innovation Place. 2022. "Lumeca Launches Canada's First Virtual Healthcare Pod." July 29, 2022. https://www.innovationplace.com/community/features/2020/07-lumeca.php.

Kates, Jennifer, Jennifer Tolbert, and Josh Michaud. "The COVID-19 'Vaccination Line': An Update on State Prioritzation Plans." Kaiser Family Foundation, January 11, 2021. https://www.kff.org/coronavirus-covid-19/issue-brief/the-covid-19-vaccination-line-an-update-on-state-prioritization-plans/.

Kaur, Harmeet. 2021. "Tribal Health Providers Have Figured Out the Keys to COVID-19 Vaccine Success. Here's Their Secret." *CNN*, February 26, 2021. https://www.cnn.com/2021/02/09/us/tribal-health-providers-covid-vaccine-trnd/index.html.

Kennedy, Ellen J. 2019. "On Indigenous Peoples Day, Recalling Forced Sterilizations of Native American Women." *MinnPost*, October 14, 2019. https://www.minnpost.com/community-voices/2019/10/on-indigenous-peoples-day-recalling-forced-sterilizations-of-native-america.

Lakhani, Nina. 2020. "Native American Tribe Takes Trailblazing Steps to Fight COVID-19 Outbreak." *The Guardian*, March 18, 2020. https://www.theguardian.com/us-news/2020/mar/18/covidcoronavirus-native-american-lummi-nation-trailblazing-steps.

Maurer, Tim, Robert Morgus, Isabel Skierka, and Mirko Hohman. 2015. "Technological Sovereignty: Missing the Point?" *2015 7th International Conference on Cyber Conflict: Architectures in Cyberspace.* Tallinn, Estonia: Institute of Electrical and Electronics Engineers: 53–68. https://doi.org/10.1109/CYCON.2015.7158468.

McFarling, Usha Lee. 2020. "'They've Been Following the Science': How the COVID-19 Pandemic Has Been Curtailed in Cherokee Nation." *STAT*, November 17, 2020. https://www.statnews.com/2020/11/17/how-covid19-has-been-curtailed-in-cherokee-nation/.

Miller, Bailey. 2021. "Tourism Closure Extended for the Remainder of 2022 on Havasupai Tribal Land Known for Waterfalls." *Fox 10 Phoenix*, June 13, 2021. https://www.fox10phoenix.com/news/tourism-closure-extended-until-june-2022-on-havasupai-tribal-land-known-for-waterfalls.

Polansky, Chris. 2021. "Cherokee Nation Opens Vaccine Eligibility to Non-Natives Living Within Reservation Boundaries." *Public Radio Tulsa*, March 10,

2021. https://www.publicradiotulsa.org/local-regional/2021-03-10/cherokee
-nation-opens-vaccine-eligibility-to-non-natives-living-within-reservation
-boundaries.

Quon, Alexander. 2021. "As Sask. Faces Growing COVID-19 Cases, Indigenous
Communities Have Charted a Different Path." *CBC News*, April 23, 2021.
https://www.cbc.ca/news/canada/saskatchewan/sask-covid-19-indigenous
-communities-1.5996026.

RedMane Technology. 2020. "A First Nation's Community Uses mCase to Help
Keep Its Residents Safe During Covid-19." May 7, 2020. https://www.red
mane.com/a-first-nations-community-uses-mcase-to-help-keep-its-residents
-safe-during-covid-19/.

Ricker, Levi. 2022. "US Supreme Court Will Not Consider Overturning Mc-
Girt Decision; Will Rule on Scope of the Landmark Ruling." *Native News
Online*, January 22, 2022. https://nativenewsonline.net/currents/us-supreme
-court-will-not-consider-overturning-mcgirt-decision-will-rule-on-scope-of
-the-landmark-ruling#.

Sanchez, Gabriel R., and Raymond Foxworth. 2021. "Native Americans and
COVID-19 Vaccine Hesitancy: Pathways Toward Increasing Vaccination Rates
for Native Communities." *HealthAffairs*, July 29, 2021. https://www.health
affairs.org/do/10.1377/forefront.20210723.390196/.

Silversmith, Shondiin. 2022. "Havasupai Tribe, at the Bottom of the Grand Canyon, Will Block Tourism Until June." *Tucson Sentinel*, January 6, 2022. https://
www.tucsonsentinel.com/local/report/010622_havasupai_tourism/havasupai
-tribe-bottom-grand-canyon-will-block-toursim-until-June.

Smith, Phillip J., David Wood, and Paul M. Darden. 2011. "Highlights of Historical Events Leading to National Surveillance of Vaccination Coverage in
the United States." *Public Health Reports* 126, no. S2: 3–12. https://doi.org/10
.1177%2F00333549111260S202.

Tatro, M. Kaye. n.d. "Curtis Act (1898)." *The Encyclopedia of Oklahoma His-
tory and Culture*. Oklahoma City, Oklahoma Historical Society. Accessed
June 26, 2023. https://www.okhistory.org/publications/enc/entry.php?entry
=CU006.

UNGA (United Nations General Assembly). 2007. Resolution 61/295, United
Nations Declaration on the Rights of Indigenous Peoples. September 13,
2007. https://www.un.org/development/desa/indigenouspeoples/wp-content
/uploads/sites/19/2018/11/UNDRIP_E_web.pdf.

Vizenor, Gerald Robert. 1999. *Manifest Manners: Narratives on Postindian Survivance*. Lincoln: University of Nebraska Press.

LEGAL RESOURCES

Cherokee Treaty, July 19, 1866 (1866)

Curtis Act, Pub. L. No. 55–517, 30 Stat. 495 (1898)

Dawes Severalty Act, Pub. L. No. 49–015, 24 Stat. 388 (1887)

Indian Removal Act, Pub. L. No. 21–148, 4 Stat. 411 (1830)

McGirt v. Oklahoma, 140 S. Ct. 2452 (2020)

Principal Chiefs Act, Pub. L. No. 91–495, 84 Stat. 1091 (1970)

Treaty of New Echota (1835)

U.N. Declaration on the Rights of Indigenous Peoples (2007)

5

THE NAVAJO NATION RESPONSE DURING THE EARLY STAGES OF THE COVID-19 PANDEMIC

MIRANDA JENSEN HASKIE

THE UNITED STATES FIRST reported the novel coronavirus on January 9, 2020, in a national newscast on *CBS News*. COVID-19, as the virus later became known, became a public health concern internationally following an outbreak in Wuhan, China. On December 1, 2019, officials from Wuhan reported high rates of a pneumonia-like illness, along with high death rates. At the time, Wuhan had the highest infection and death rates worldwide. The United States then reported the first coronavirus death of a man in Washington state on January 21, 2020 (Teichner 2020).

The first case of COVID-19 on the Navajo Nation was reported March 16, 2020, in the community of Chilchinbeto, Arizona, but within another month, the number had risen to over a thousand. The first Navajo death was reported March 24, 2020. By April 17, 2020, the Navajo Department of Health (NDOH) had reported 1,127 cases of COVID-19, with 44 confirmed deaths, placing the Navajo Nation COVID-19 death rate at nearly 4 percent. The Navajo Nation reported 3,204 cases of COVID-19, and deaths numbered 102 on May 11, 2020. By May 17, 2020, about two months after the initial March 16 COVID-19 case, there were 4,002 cases of COVID-19 on the Navajo Nation, with 140 reported deaths. On February 22, 2021, there were 29,531 positive cases with 1,145 confirmed deaths (NDOH 2023).

This chapter reports on an observational study in one small Navajo Nation community about the use of personal safety measures during the height of the COVID-19 pandemic.

NAVAJO NATION COVID-19
RATES AND RESPONSES

Upon examination, the COVID-19 rates on the Navajo Nation were alarming. The Navajo Nation worked independently of but in concert with state health agencies in addressing the pandemic. The Navajo Nation spans three states in Arizona, New Mexico, and Utah. One example of state action occurred when Michelle Lujan Grisham, New Mexico's governor, held a statewide news conference on March 11, 2020, in which she declared a public health emergency. Governor Lujan Grisham informed the public about New Mexico's measures to contain the virus (Office of Governor Michelle Lujan Grisham 2020). Some measures resulted in the cancellation of public events, including the Gathering of Nations powwow held in Albuquerque, New Mexico, an annual spring event attracting nearly 100,000 people, including many Navajo Nation citizens.

By April 20, 2020, *NBC News* reported that rates of COVID-19 on the Navajo Nation ranked third highest in the country, following New York and New Jersey (McFadden et al. 2020). By May 11, 2020, the Navajo Nation was reported to have the highest per capita rates of COVID-19 in the United States; these rates far outpaced the rates in New York and New Jersey (Baek 2020).

One infection-control practice involves the prescriptive use of personal protective equipment (PPE) (WHO, n.d.). The author conducted a study to observe public use of PPE in one Navajo Nation community, Lukachukai, during April 2020 and from January 21 through February 4, 2021. This study set out to observe which populations within this community exhibited the greatest use of PPE and which populations exhibited the lowest use of PPE in protection against COVID-19.

NAVAJO NATION POPULATION

Romero (2021; U.S. Census Bureau 2020c) reported the Navajo Nation as the largest tribe in the United States, with an enrollment of 399,494 people. According to the U.S. Census Bureau (2020b), the total population reported within reservation boundary was 165,168; this reflected a 3 percent decrease in reservation population between 2010 and 2020.

The Navajo Nation population aged 65 and over make up 13 percent, 30 percent are youth ages 19 and under, and the remaining 57 percent are adults ages 20 to 64 (U.S. Census Bureau 2021b). The total population in the community of Lukachukai, Arizona, was 1,637, with 100 percent reported as Native American (U.S. Census 2021a). Population by gender was 50 percent male and 50 percent female (U.S. Census Bureau 2021a).

Lukachukai is one of 110 chapter communities located on the 27,000-square-mile reservation of the Navajo Nation (Navajo Nation, n.d.; Navajo Nation 2023b). There are two stores, one of which was the location of this observational study. The store serves as a grocery store and also houses the United States Postal Service office, playing a vital role in community life. On any given day, Navajo from different gender, age, and socioeconomic demographics frequent the store to collect mail and/or purchase consumable goods, providing a cross-sectional representation of Lukachukai community members.

NAVAJO NATION "STAY-AT-HOME ORDER" AND WEEKEND LOCKDOWN

There were fourteen COVID-19 cases among the on-reservation population of the Navajo Nation on March 19, 2020 (NDOH 2023). In response, on March 20, 2020, Navajo Nation then president Jonathan Nez issued Public Health Emergency Order No. 2020–003, colloquially referred to as a "stay-at-home-order" (NDOH 2020). Stay-at-home orders were already in place in many jurisdictions across the United States and the Navajo Nation followed suit. By April 10, 2020, there were 597 cases of COVID-19 on the Navajo Nation, with 22 reported deaths (NDOH 2023). As COVID-19 infection and death rates continued to rise on the Navajo Nation, on April 5, 2020, President Nez issued Public Health Emergency Order No. 2020–005, a "57-hour curfew weekend" that ran from Friday, April 10, at 8:00 p.m. through 5:00 a.m. on Monday, April 13, 2020 (Silverman 2020). There were 35 public health orders issued for weekend lockdowns between April 10, 2020, and January 22, 2021 (NDOH 2023). Those in violation could be fined $1,000 and/or ordered to serve 30 days in jail. Becenti (2020) reported 825 criminal nuisance citations and 480 traffic stops between April 10 and May 10, 2020.

PERSONAL PROTECTIVE EQUIPMENT

Personal protective equipment (PPE) includes masks (N95 or non-N95), handkerchiefs or cloth coverings to protect one's nose and mouth, disposable gloves, and protective eyewear other than prescription glasses. Wearing a mask and disposable gloves greatly reduces the risk of contracting COVID-19 (Núñez et al. 2020).

Utilizing PPE is an effective infection control practice that can also reduce the transmission of COVID-19 by asymptomatic carriers (Sohrabi et al. 2020), whose capacity to spread the virus puts the public at greater risk (Feng et al. 2020). In their interim guidance in the earliest days of the pandemic, the World Health Organization did not recommend PPE for public use (Moore, Bouchoucha, and Buchwald 2021, 709). By March 2020, public health officials had readily altered practices in response to the changing nature of how COVID-19 was being contracted (WHO 2020).

The Centers for Disease Control and Prevention (CDC) guidelines for wearing face masks and utilizing other PPE worked to change public practices to prevent the spread of the coronavirus (Moore, Bouchoucha, and Buchwald 2021, 709). By promoting these safety guidelines, the CDC acted with transparency and avoided the consequences of "public misinformation" about the virus, which can delay the development of prevention measures and lead to "racism, incorrect public precautions, and unprecedented fear surrounding COVID-19" (Sohrabi et al. 2020, 10).

On April 17, 2020, the NDOH issued Public Health Emergency Order No. 2020–007 mandating use of masks in public due to COVID-19, defining "public" as any area outside the home where someone could come within six feet of a person not from their household. The public health emergency order also advised handwashing with soap for twenty seconds or using 60 percent alcohol-based hand sanitizer when water and soap were unavailable; disinfecting frequently touched surfaces in the home; not touching one's face, nose, eyes, or mouth; and avoiding all public gatherings and unnecessary travel (NDOH 2020).

STUDY METHODS

This study was conducted by randomly observing Lukachukai community members waiting in line to enter the store. While in a personal vehicle outside the store, this researcher observed the population for two safety measures—use of PPE and the practice of social distancing. The researcher observed mixed groups of male and female community members from a variety of age groups. The people observed included 49 percent males and 51 percent females. Based on the 2020 census (U.S. Census Bureau 2020a), this data offered a representative sample. In total, there were 200 community members observed. The groups of community members were observed every day of the week, Monday through Friday, at 2:00 pm daily. This particular time was chosen because this was when people often came in to collect daily mail. The researcher observed the groups without any interference, and community members were unaware that they were being observed.

RESULTS

Overall, 200 observations were conducted. In the first observational study, the population included 100 people in the sample, with 50 males and 50 females. The data presented in figures 5.1 and 5.2 are from the first 100 people observed. A discussion about the second group of 100 people observed follows. Throughout the chapter, the terms *Navajo* and *Diné* are used interchangeably. The primary goal of the observational study was to examine the differences among Lukachukai community members and their utilization of PPE to protect against contracting COVID-19. Figure 5.1 exhibits data collected over the first 10-day study, in which the general population was observed utilizing PPE while waiting in line in front of the store.

The majority of people observed, 59 percent, were wearing PPE, including face coverings (N95 masks or cloth coverings), gloves (either on one hand or both hands), and/or protective eye covering. Once during the initial 10-day study, a Navajo male was also observed wearing a protective eye covering similar to the plastic eye glasses worn by construction workers. More Navajo females wore PPE, at 53 percent (31 of the 59), while 47 percent (28 of the 59) of Navajo males wore PPE. Becenti (2020) reported on May 13, 2020, that "the average COVID-positive Diné is 44 and there are 1,594 men and 1,798 women who've tested positive. As for confirmed deaths the average age is 65 and more men have succumbed to the illness compared to females with 72 men and 47 women deceased."

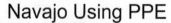

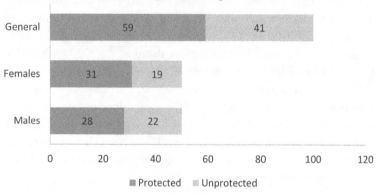

FIGURE 5.1 Navajo PPE use. Graph by author.

Data on the percentage of Navajo wearing PPE by estimated age group (based on the researcher's knowledge of the community members) was also collected. Those age 19 or younger totaled 5 in the sample, 26 were in the age group 20–29, 24 were in the age group 30–39, 8 were in the age group 40–49, 12 were in the age group 50–59, 12 were in the age group 60–69, and 13 were age 70 and older.

According to the data in the observational study, the age group least likely to wear PPE was the age group 40–49. The data was stark enough to correlate with the average age of 44 for Navajo Nation COVID-19 cases. The age groups of 30–39 and 50–59 were those most likely to be wearing PPE. The age groups of 40–49 and 20–29 were those least likely to be wearing PPE. Based on observational data, more Navajo males were less likely to wear PPE.

Figure 5.2 provides data on the daily use of PPE over the first 10-day observational study. On any given day, at least 50 percent of the Navajo visiting the post office / store in the community of Lukachukai were observed to be wearing PPE.

At the beginning of the study, people in line at the store were not practicing social distancing of six feet between each person. However, on April 17, 2020, a considerable difference was noticed and people were found to be practicing the required social distancing. As mentioned earlier, the Navajo Public Health Emergency Order No. 2020–007 was passed on

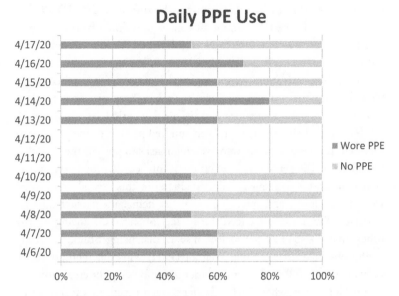

FIGURE 5.2 Daily PPE use. Graph by author.

the same day. Painted red lines six feet apart were observed on the ground, and customers distanced themselves accordingly. This social distancing was not by choice; it was imposed by the store owner per the public health emergency order.

The researcher noted the store owner's additional measures to ensure public safety the following week. On April 20, 2020, the store owner would periodically stand outside and remind people not wearing a mask, "When you come in here, you're supposed to have a mask," and if they proceeded to enter without one, the store owner reminded them, "You need to get a mask," at which point one customer left the store. The researcher rolled down the car window to hear the store owner's instructions. On April 20 and thereafter, all customers had to wear a mask to enter the store. Following the store requirement, on April 20, 90 percent of customers were observed wearing PPE—some kind of cloth mask or simply a handkerchief. A very few were observed wearing the blue surgical masks worn by medical workers. During the time of observation, only that one customer without PPE was told to leave the store. The owner had to close the store from December 18, 2020, through January 2, 2021, despite the store's best efforts to prevent the spread of COVID-19. The store owners informed the community that some of their family members had tested positive for COVID-19 and they had to close in compliance with the recommended 14 days of isolation following exposure.

In all, 200 observations were completed. Data presented in this section were from the first 100 observations. The researcher carried out a second group of 100 observations over another 10-day period, from January 21, 2021, through February 4, 2021. One hundred percent of the people observed in this second group were wearing masks to prevent the spread of COVID-19. The gender representation of this second group was 46 percent male and 54 percent female. Again, all in this second group were wearing face masks and practicing social distancing. The researcher found when the line leader practiced the six feet of social distancing, all the others in line also practiced six feet of social distancing. Studies on group conformity by Asch (1952) and Milgram (1964) help explain how ordinary individuals will follow the lead in order to avoid being different from the group. Conversely, when the line leader did not practice six feet of social distancing, the others in line only sporadically practiced social distancing.

DISCUSSION AND IMPLICATIONS

This study provides insight about PPE use in one community on the vast Navajo Nation reservation as COVID-19 rates reached frightening levels. More Navajo women were found to be using PPE compared to Navajo men, across all age groups. The age group of 40–49 was least likely to be wearing PPE based on this observational study, which correlates to the average age of 44 for COVID-19 cases among Navajo (Becenti 2020). The NDOH reported the average age of death from COVID-19 was 66, with the majority being Navajo males. On May 5, 2020, the NDOH reported 79 deaths since the onset of the pandemic, which included 48 Navajo males and 31 females. The mortality rate for Navajo men on May 5, 2020, was higher despite the fact that more Navajo females (1,368) had tested COVID-19 positive compared to the 1,191 Navajo males. On February 22, 2021, Navajo males under the age of 30 through ages 70–79 had higher mortality rates than females in these age groups. In contrast, Navajo females experienced higher infection and mortality rates in the age group 80 and above (NDOH 2023). This shift can be explained by longevity among female populations, as is true in the population of Navajo females. When 1,000 Navajo had died by January 28, 2021, Becenti (2021) reported that two-thirds of the deaths were among Navajo ages 65 and over.

In the first group of 100 observed, more Navajo females wore PPE, yet this demographic more broadly still had a higher number who tested positive. One factor that may explain this is that Navajo females are primary caretakers of family members. Even though Navajo males experienced higher COVID-19 mortality rates, Schrank et al.'s study sheds light on the link between female caregivers and their overall health. Females are "reported to spend more hours caring . . . and less often draw on support by other family members or professional services" (2016, 808). On the Navajo Nation, the same is true—females are the primary caregivers for sick family members. Valentina Blackhorse, former Miss Western Navajo, succumbed from COVID-19 after caring for her COVID-19 positive boyfriend. At first, she and her baby daughter both tested negative. Despite her family's urging her to stay at their family home with her daughter, she told her family "she's going to take care of her boyfriend" (Allen 2020). At the time of her passing, she was only 28 years old, leaving a daughter behind. This case is one example demonstrating how easily caregivers of COVID-19 patients can contract the virus.

Moreover, American Indians and Alaskan Natives (AI/ANs) are considered a high-risk health group. AI/ANs have higher rates of diabetes, high blood pressure, heart disease, obesity, and other chronic diseases like cancer (Denny et al. 2005). The CDC (2022) reported higher risk of mortality by COVID-19 among populations with serious underlying health conditions, including racial and ethnic minority populations.

The lack of running water for 30 percent of Navajo living on the reservation can be a significant compounding issue during a public health crisis such as COVID-19, where running water is required for safety measures such as washing one's hands (Baek 2020; Lee 2020; McFadden et al. 2020). The Navajo Nation's housing insecurity further contributes to the difficulty in containing the spread of COVID-19. In tribal areas, more than 16 percent of AI/ANs reported overcrowded housing, according to U.S. Housing and Urban Development standards (Pindus et al. 2017); thus, the Navajo Nation also experiences housing insecurity. Multigenerational households, like many on the Navajo Nation, had a greater incidence of spreading COVID-19 when one household member tested COVID-19 positive (Michener et al. 2020). Additionally, an IHS (n.d.) fact sheet described AI/AN populations as having "inadequate education, disproportionate poverty, discrimination in the delivery of health services, and cultural differences. These are broad quality of life issues rooted in economic adversity and poor social conditions." These sociocultural factors exacerbate Navajo patient diagnosis, care, and treatment of COVID-19.

LIMITATIONS OF STUDY

There are several limitations to this observational study. One limitation is that such a study cannot examine the causes for why some persons did not wear PPE. Second, the age ranges were estimated based on the researcher's knowledge of fellow community members. As well, the data presented are not representative of the entire Navajo Nation on-reservation population. Rather, this observational study was compiled in one community on the Navajo Nation. Again, the Navajo Nation is situated in three states including Arizona, New Mexico, and Utah. In future studies, observational data collection should be followed up with a questionnaire for research participants to discover why they were not wearing PPE.

CONCLUSIONS

The present study, along with other research into health disparities, suggests the need for strategies to address the continuing impact of COVID-19 as well as future contagious disease–related public health emergencies affecting the Navajo Nation. Strategies should include disseminating more public health information, educating the Navajo Nation public about COVID-19, distributing PPE to members of the Navajo Nation, and addressing water and housing insecurity. The dissemination of public health information can embrace all forms of formal and social media utilized by the Navajo Nation, including KTNN AM radio station, Facebook, Instagram, newspapers such as the *Navajo Times*, and public health pamphlets.

Regular communication with the public is necessary to mitigate the spread of COVID-19 (Sohrabi et al. 2020).

While the dissemination of information about COVID-19 can assist, the Navajo Nation still requires more public health education about COVID-19, particularly about prevention practices such as using PPE, social distancing measures, disinfecting frequently, testing, symptom identification, and protocols for treatment. The combination of these measures can mitigate the spread of COVID-19. On the other hand, the reality is that a lack of running water, along with the Navajo Nation poverty rate of 37.5 percent (U.S. Census Bureau 2021c), housing insecurity, and chronic health conditions, make containing COVID-19 difficult.

At the outset, President Jonathan Nez and his cabinet successfully led a unified and coordinated effort to mitigate the spread of COVID-19 on the Navajo Nation. President Nez and Vice President Myron Lizer hosted weekly town hall meetings on YouTube to keep the public informed. These meetings were held in the Navajo language to reach elderly Navajo populations and others fluent in the Navajo language, and to convey Navajo cultural teachings. Ramona Antone-Nez, director of the Navajo Epidemiology Center (NEC), and NEC staff reported the COVID-19 data on their website in coordination with Dr. Jill Jim, NDOH executive director. The NEC provided a model database that presented daily updates on COVID-19 numbers. Antone-Nez (2021) presented at the Emerging Infection and Tribal Communities Conference hosted by Diné College. She explained how the Navajo Nation already had built partnerships and were in close communication with the states of Arizona, New Mexico, and Utah departments of health as they were watching COVID-19 come closer to the Navajo Nation. The NEC and NDOH had built these partnerships years in advance. They told Navajo Nation leaders they were confident in this relationship and that these state health departments would inform the Navajo Nation when the first Navajo COVID-19 positive case was diagnosed so the Navajo Nation could tell their story. Antone-Nez (2021) also reported that in response to COVID-19, the NDOH had issued thirty-two public health emergency orders in 2020 and three public health emergency orders in 2021. These public health emergency orders included the stay-at-home orders to prevent further spread of COVID-19. These orders along with the partnerships with state health departments, NEC's COVID-19 database, the weekly town hall meetings, social media posts, COVID-19 vaccine drives, and the unified leadership of President Nez and his cabinet were successful measures in the mitigation of COVID-19 and therefore may offer insight into best practices for future public health emergencies.

REFERENCES

Allen, Krista. 2020. "COVID Claims Former Miss Western, 28." *Navajo Times*, April 26, 2020. https://navajotimes.com/reznews/covid-claims-former-miss -western-28/.

Antone-Nez, Ramona. 2021. "Working Together: Feds, States, Tribal Communities; Sharing Epidemiological Data." February 18, 2021. Paper presented at the virtual Emerging Infection and Tribal Communities Conference, hosted by Diné College, Tsaile, AZ. https://www.dinecollege.edu/wp-content/uploads /2021/02/Presentation5-RamonaAntoneNez-021921.pdf.

Arizona Rural Policy Institute. 2010. *Demographic Analysis of the Navajo Nation Using 2010 Census and 2010 American Community Survey Estimates*. Flagstaff: W. A. Franke College of Business, Northern Arizona University. https://in .nau.edu/wp-content/uploads/sites/156/2018/12/navajo_nation_0.pdf.

Ash, Solomon. 1952. *Social Psychology*. Englewood Cliffs, NJ: Prentice-Hall.

Baek, Grace. 2020. "Navajo Nation Residents Face Coronavirus Without Running Water." *CBS News*, May 8, 2020. https://www.cbsnews.com/news/corona virus-navajo-nation-running-water-cbsn-originals/.

Becenti, Arlyssa. 2020. "COVID Death Toll Spikes; Cases Near 4,000." *Navajo Times*, May 13, 2020. https://navajotimes.com/coronavirus-updates/covid-death -toll-spikes-cases-near-4000/.

Becenti, Arlyssa. 2021. "COVID Deaths Reach 1,000 on Navajo Nation." *Navajo Times*, January 28, 2021. https://navajotimes.com/reznews/covid-deaths-reach -1000-on-navajo-nation/.

CDC (Centers for Disease Control and Prevention). 2022. "People Who Need to Take Extra Precautions." Last updated August 11, 2022. https://www.cdc.gov /coronavirus/2019-ncov/need-extra-precautions/index.html.

Denny, Clark H., Deborah Holtzman, R. Turner Goins, and Janet B. Croft. 2005. "Disparities in Chronic Disease Factors and Health Status Between American Indian/Alaska Native and White Elders: Findings from a Telephone Survey, 2001 and 2002." *American Journal of Public Health* 95, no. 5 (May) 825–27. https://doi.org/10.2105/ajph.2004.043489.

Feng, Shuo, Chen Shen, Nan Xia, Wei Song, Mengzhen Fan, and Benjamin J. Cowling. 2020. "Rational Use of Face Masks in the COVID-19 Pandemic."

LANCET Respiratory Medicine 8, no. 5: 434–36. https://doi.org/10.1016/S2213
-2600(20)30134-X.

IHS (Indian Health Service). n.d.. "Fact Sheets: Disparities." Accessed May 15,
2020. https://www.ihs.gov/newsroom/factsheets/disparities/.

Lee, Kurtis. 2020. "No Running Water. No Electricity. On Navajo Nation, Coronavirus Creates Worry and Confusion as Cases Surge." *Los Angeles Times*,
March 29, 2020. https://www.latimes.com/world-nation/story/2020-03-29/no
-running-water-no-electricity-in-navajo-nation-coronavirus-creates-worry
-and-confusion-as-cases-surge.

McFadden, Cynthia, Jaime Longoria, Christine Romo, and Kenzi Abou-Sabe.
2020. "Coronavirus Batters the Navajo Nation, and It's About to Get Worse."
Today Show, April 20, 2020. https://www.today.com/health/coronavirus-batters
-navajo-nation-it-s-about-get-worse-t179219?cid=eml_tdb_20200420.

Michener, Lloyd, Sergio Aguilar-Gaxiola, Philip M. Alberti, Manuel J. Casta-
neda, Brian C. Castrucci, Lisa Macon Harrison, Lauren S. Hughes, Al Richmond, and Nina Wallerstein. 2020. "Engaging With Communities—Lessons
(Re)Learned From COVID-19." *Prevention of Chronic Diseases* 17, E65 (July):
1–8. http://dx.doi.org/10.5888/pcd17.200250.

Milgram, Stanley. 1964. "Group Pressure and Action Against a Person." *Journal
of Abnormal and Social Psychology* 69, no. 2: 137–43. https://psycnet.apa.org/doi
/10.1037/h0047759.

Moore, Kathleen A., Stéphane L. Bouchoucha, and Petra Buchwald. 2021. "A Comparison of the Public's Use of PPE and Strategies to Avoid Contagion During
the COVID-19 Pandemic in Australia and Germany." *Nursing and Health Sciences* 23, no. 3: 708–14. https://doi-org.fgul.idm.oclc.org/10.1111/nhs.12857.

Navajo Nation. n.d. "Navajo Nation Chapter Directory Listing." Accessed July 28,
2023. https://docs.google.com/spreadsheets/d/19pHQM1NK5gB6ky_uS7Bne
3fkPDkEhqqyxDerTMqtmYI/edit#gid=0.

Navajo Nation. 2023. "History." https://www.navajo-nsn.gov/History.

NDOH (Navajo Department of Health). 2020. Public Health Emergency Order No. 2020–007. Navajo Office of Environmental Health & Protection
Program. April 17, 2020. https://ndoh.navajo-nsn.gov/Portals/0/COVID-19/
News/NDOH%20Public%20Health%20Emergency%20Order%202020-007
%20Dikos%20Ntsaaigii-19.pdf.

NDOH (Navajo Department of Health). 2023. "Dikos Ntsaaigii-19 (COVID-19)."
Last updated May 4, 2023. https://www.ndoh.navajo-nsn.gov/COVID-19.

NEC (Navajo Epidemiology Center). 2013. *Navajo Population Profile 2010 U.S.
Census*. Window Rock, AZ: Navajo Department of Health. https://nec.navajo
-nsn.gov/Portals/0/Reports/NN2010PopulationProfile.pdf.

Núñez, Ana, Maria Madison, Renata Schiavo, Ronit Elk, and Holly G. Prigerson. 2020. "Responding to Healthcare Disparities and Challenges with Access to Care During COVID-19." *Health Equity* 14, no. 4: 117–28. https://doi.org/10.1089/heq.2020.29000.rtl.

Office of Governor Michelle Lujuan Grisham. 2020. "Updated: Department of Health Announce First Positive COVID-19 Cases in New Mexico." Press release. March 11, 2020. https://www.governor.state.nm.us/2020/03/11/updated-governor-department-of-health-announce-first-positive-covid-19-cases-in-new-mexico/.

Pindus, Nancy, G. Thomas Kingsley, Jennifer Biess, Diane Levy, Jasmine Simington, and Christopher Hayes. 2017. *Housing Needs of American Indians and Alaska Natives in Tribal Areas: A Report from the Assessment of American Indian, Alaska Native and Native Hawaiian Housing Needs.* Washington, D.C.: U.S. Department of Housing and Urban Development, Office of Policy Development and Research. https://www.huduser.gov/portal/publications/Housing NeedsAmerIndians-ExecSumm.html.

Romero, Simon. 2021. "The Navajo Nation Becomes Largest Tribe in U.S. After Pandemic Enrollment Surge." *New York Times*, May 21, 2021. https://www.nytimes.com/2021/05/21/us/navajo-cherokee-population.html.

Schrank, Beate, Alexandra Ebert-Vogel, Michaela Amering, Eva K. Masel, Marie Neubauer, Herbert Watzke, Sonja Zehetmayer, and Sophie Schur. 2016. "Gender Differences in Caregiver Burden and Its Determinants in Family Members of Terminally Ill Cancer Patients." *Psycho-Oncology* 25, no. 7: 808–14. https://doi.org/10.1002/pon.4005.

Silverman, Hollie. 2020. "The Navajo Nation Is Under a Weekend Curfew to Help Combat the Spread of Coronavirus." *CNN*, April 12, 2020. https://edition.cnn.com/2020/04/12/us/navajo-nation-coronavirus/index.html.

Sohrabi, Catrin, Zaid Alsafi, Niamh O'Neill, Mehdi Khan, Ahmed Kerwan, Ahmed Al-Jabir, Christos Iosifidls, and Riaz Agha. 2020. "World Health Organization Declares Global Emergency: A Review of the 2019 Novel Coronavirus (COVID-19)." *International Journal of Surgery* 76 (April): 71–76. https://doi.org/10.1016/j.ijsu.2020.02.034.

Teichner, Martha. 2020. "Cover Story: Why Wasn't America Ready?" *CBS News*, April 26, 2020. https://www.cbsnews.com/news/this-week-on-sunday-morning-april-26-2020/.

U.S. Census Bureau. 2020a. "2020 Census Population of Lukachukai, AZ." https://data.census.gov/profile?g=160XX00US0442660.

U.S. Census Bureau. 2020b. "Navajo Nation Reservation Population." https://data.census.gov/profile?g=2500000US2430.

U.S. Census Bureau. 2020c. "Total Navajo Nation Population." https://www
.census.gov/search-results.html?searchType=web&cssp=SERP&q=Navajo
%20Nation%20Reservation%20and%20Off-Reservation%20Trust%20Land,
%20AZ--NM--UT.

U.S. Census Bureau. 2021a. "American Community Survey: Lukachukai Population." https://censusreporter.org/profiles/16000US0442660-lukachukai-az/.

U.S. Census Bureau. 2021b. "American Community Survey: Navajo Nation Population by Age." https://data.census.gov/table?g=2500000US2430&tid=ACSS
T5Y2021.S0101.

U.S. Census Bureau. 2021c. "Navajo Nation Reservation and Off-Reservation
Trust Land, AZ-NM-UT: Poverty Status in the Past 12 Months, American Community Survey 5-Year Estimates." https://www.census.gov/tribal/
?aianihh=2430.

WHO (World Health Organization). n.d. "Coronavirus Disease (COVID-19)
Advice for the Public: When and How to Use Masks." Last updated December 2021. https://www.who.int/emergencies/diseases/novel-coronavirus-2019
/advice-for-public/when-and-how-to-use-masks.

6

MEDIA FRAMING OF THE COVID-19 PANDEMIC ACROSS NATIVE NATIONS

STEFANIE KUNZE AND EARLENE CAMARILLO

ON DECEMBER 10, 2021, Navajo Nation president Jonathan Nez urged the Navajo Nation to "not let down our guard during this holiday season. We've seen how quickly variants can spread in our communities, especially during family gatherings" (Associated Press 2021). Nez cautioned that the tribe's health-care system could not afford another surge. This dire warning came roughly two years after the unprecedented novel coronavirus (COVID-19) pandemic began sweeping the globe, with the resulting respiratory infections highlighting social, ethnic and racial, political, and economic inequalities worldwide. As the COVID-19 pandemic rapidly became a global crisis, it dominated national media headlines in the United States, where the Navajo Nation and other Indigenous communities were hit disproportionately hard by the pandemic with case numbers outstripping surrounding areas. However, stories covering its impact on Indigenous communities were relatively scarce among national news outlets. While it is not uncommon for Indigenous perspectives to be absent from these sources (Campisteguy, Heilbronner, and Nakamura-Rybak 2018; Leavitt et al. 2015; Moore and Lanthorn 2017), this absence is problematic since public understanding of a topic as important is directly shaped by whether and how much media coverage a topic receives (McCombs 2005; McCombs, Shaw, and Weaver 2014). One area of particular distinction in how the national media focuses on Indigenous topics is the topic of resilience. Resilience, which we will discuss in more depth later, emphasizes the ability of Indigenous Peoples to not just merely survive, as so often presented in Western approaches, but to thrive under challenging and hostile circumstances stemming from Western colonization. This resilience, or survivance, has become a particular focus in Indigenous research.[1] In this chapter, however, we specifically examine media coverage of the pandemic, paying particular attention to the extent of coverage and how the stories were framed.

CONTEXTUALIZING COVID-19'S IMPACT ON INDIGENOUS NATIONS

We have seen widely differing political decisions at the local, state, Native nation, and federal levels within the United States, which continued to lead the world in COVID-19 mortality rates as of March 2023 (CRC, n.d.). Decisions at state levels were frequently at odds with federal guidelines, and local and tribal decisions often stood in contrast to executive orders from state governors. It is important to remember that, except in the few states where Public Law 280 applies (Alaska, California, Minnesota, Nebraska, Oregon, and Wisconsin), state governments have no decision-making powers over Indigenous reservation or trust land; Native nations are sovereign, domestic dependent nations, as defined by Chief Justice John Marshall in the 1831 Supreme Court case *Cherokee Nation v. Georgia* (Bens 2020), and hold a unique relationship with the federal government. Therefore, decisions at the Native nation level, so-called minor legislation (Turner 2005), sometimes stand in stark contrast to those of the surrounding states. See, for example, the case in South Dakota where Governor Kristi Noem clashed with the Oglala Lakota Nation and Cheyenne River Sioux Tribe over roadblocks that the Sioux Nation erected to prevent outsiders from entering sovereign Sioux land in an effort to minimize exposure to COVID-19 (O'Brien 2020). Similarly, the Navajo Nation

---

1. In a discussion on this topic at the Western Social Science Association's 2022 conference, people in the audience who represented different tribes across the country noted that, at the beginning of the pandemic, they turned to their elders and those within the community who hold traditional knowledge for ways to protect themselves and their families against this new disease. These stories represent additional interpretations of resilience from Indigenous people.

government, among other Indigenous nations in Arizona, prominently put the Navajo Nation and its five agencies on curfews and lockdowns, effectively limiting enrolled Diné in coming and going. Highlighting the differences in governance between Indigenous nations and settler-state governments, Navajo Nation decisions could not be more different from the actions that Arizona governor Doug Ducey took, avoiding statewide mask mandates and prohibiting local jurisdictions from imposing their own mask mandates (Bowing 2020; Innes 2020; Martinez 2022). In some cases, these situations rekindled existing conflicts tied to tribal sovereignty and states' rights, as the South Dakota example illustrates.

The U.S. federal government is constitutionally obligated to provide for and support *federally recognized tribes* (Conner, Fryar, and Johnson 2017; Deloria 2010; Jewell 2014), including providing health care to tribal members (NCAI 2020; Warne and Frizzel 2014); however, the federal government fell short in these responsibilities, even with the passage of the Coronavirus Aid, Relief, and Economic Security (CARES) Act on March 27, 2020 and implementation thereafter (van Dorn et al. 2000). After the CARES Act was passed, the allocated aid for federally recognized tribes was withheld for weeks (Cancryn 2020; Klemko 2020; Lakhani 2020b) and, in some cases, required judicial orders to disburse funds (Beitsch 2020; Fonseca 2020). According to reporting and social media posts, deliveries and help from the Federal Emergency Management Agency and the National Guard were delayed or misguided (Diethelm 2020; Joe 2020; Ortiz 2020). This adds to a long history of settler colonialism, during which Indigenous communities have been reduced, removed and terminated, marginalized, and disproportionately affected by the spread of new contagious diseases (Emerson and Montoya 2021; Jones 2006; Leggat-Barr, Uchikoshi, and Goldman 2021; Power et al. 2020). The U.S. government's neglect of its trust responsibility to Indigenous nations, which stipulates that "the federal government has a legal and moral obligation to provide for the well-being of American Indians through the provision of such services as education and health care, and to respect the rights of tribes to self-govern" (Conner, Fryar, and Johnson 2017, 57), becomes particularly visible during times of crisis. The withholding and slow disbursement of aid was reminiscent of prior interactions with the settler-colonial federal government, and the coronavirus pandemic is adding to this legacy.

Many Native American nations were initially hit particularly hard by the pandemic, yet data collection, which is important for clearly understanding the nature of a problem and developing solutions, was severely lacking. Early reports showed that in Arizona, for example, that Indigenous residents in the state made up 18 percent of COVID-19 deaths by May 2020 even though they only represented 5.3 percent of the state population (Tai et al. 2021). By March 2021, data indicated that American Indians and Alaska Natives (AI/ANs) were dying from COVID-19 at 2 to 2.4 times the rate of non-Hispanic white Americans (Burki 2021; Qeadan et al. 2021). One study used a comprehensive approach to assembling mortality data and places the COVID-19 mortality rate of Native Americans in 2020 at "2.8 times as high as among Whites and is considerably higher than the corresponding values of 1.6 and 1.8 for Black and Latino populations" (Leggat-Barr, Uchikoshi, and Goldman 2021, 1196). This data is not broken down by Native nation but rather is all-encompassing of the AI/AN population. The Indian Health Service (IHS) breaks down its COVID-19 data by IHS areas: there are eleven areas and data are reported from "tribal and urban Indian organization facilities" and programs (IHS 2023). Despite severe lockdowns on some Native American reservations, Leggat-Barr, Uchikoshi, and Goldman's study suggests "that these advantages may be outweighed by the many risk factors for COVID-19 infection and severity that are disproportionately present on reservations" (2021, 6), since, across the United States, "strong policy responses, such as lockdowns of businesses, restrictions on size of gatherings and travel, border closures, and quarantines have been associated with reduced COVID-19 transmission" (2021, 1188).

When specifically looking at scholarly and news articles covering COVID-19 on Indigenous lands, it is clear that during the time period in which we examined media for this project (January 1, 2020–September 30, 2020), coverage was limited and data and peer-reviewed research corroborating the information reported in these news articles were even scarcer. The first COVID-19 case in the United States reportedly was detected in January 2020 on the Lummi Reservation in Washington State (Lakhani 2020a). On the Navajo Nation, cases were reported by March 17, 2020 (Abou-Sabe et al. 2020; Emerson and Montoya 2021), and on the Choctaw reservation by "mid-March" (Walker 2020b). The Navajo Nation (the Diné people) "garnered considerable media attention" (Leggat-Barr,

Uchikoshi, and Goldman 2021, 5), whereas reports from other Indigenous communities are notably missing from this time frame, and the total frequency of articles referencing infections among Native Americans is extremely limited. The Navajo Nation's struggle with COVID-19 became a "fad" in the media, which aligns with research that suggests that certain issues "occasionally (e.g., during the Red Power era) provide American Indians with an attentive national audience" (Deloria 1986, 203; Turner 2005, 16).

By April 10, 2020, however, a study concluded that COVID-19 infections per Native American reservation averaged three, yet, "at the extreme end, the Navajo Nation had already registered" approximately 599 COVID-19 cases. The same study also identified that the infection rate of COVID-19 was "more than 4 times higher" for on-reservation populations than the general U.S. population (Rodriguez-Lonebear et al. 2020, 374). While a comprehensive overview of infection rates by Native American nations is not publicly available, by October 2021, the IHS (2023) stated on its website that "American Indians and Alaska Natives have infection rates over 3.5 times higher than non-Hispanic whites, are over four times more likely to be hospitalized as a result of COVID-19, and have higher rates of mortality at younger ages than non-Hispanic whites." Infections on tribal nations are represented in the eleven IHS areas or included in county statistics, and perhaps both. A total of 7,683 AI/ANs were recorded as having passed away from COVID-19 by October 2021 (NIHB, n.d.). Many Indigenous websites do not feature COVID-19 statistics or provide only limited case information. As a case example, in October 2021, the Navajo Department of Health shared a total of 35,583 COVID-19, or Dikos Ntsaaígíí-19 in Diné bizaad (Navajo language), cases but no cumulative positivity rate (NDOH 2023). Native Americans were clearly being hit harder than surrounding communities, with an average "cumulative percent positive" rate of 8.9 percent across IHS areas (IHS 2023), and yet, the national media did not begin reporting on Native American vulnerability until infections reached exponential growth on tribal land, even while the coronavirus was central to media reporting more generally. The *New York Times* (the *Times*) did not publish anything on Native Americans until early April, when it was undeniable that Indigenous nations were being disproportionately impacted (Eisenberg 2020; Lakhani 2020b; Sottile and Ortiz 2020; Klar 2020).

Despite these reported disproportional mortality rates, Native American nations received limited national news attention. For example, the Associated Press, which is generally regarded as an unbiased source of information and a source for content for many national news agencies, published 145 articles on COVID-19 and related issues between January 1, 2020, and September 30, 2020. Of those articles, only 32 (22 percent) focused on Native Americans. Similarly, Reuters, another well-regarded news source, published 139 articles, of which only 11 (8 percent) touched on Native American topics. During this time frame, the COVID-19 pandemic was the topic of practically all front-page news; however, proportionally to the U.S. total population, Indigenous nations were severely underrepresented. The five Navajo Nation agencies specifically, were experiencing infection rates far outpacing rates in surrounding counties and states (Eisenberg 2020; Lakhani 2021; Sottile and Ortiz 2020; Klar 2020; Powell 2020) and were garnering a majority of the mainstream media attention focused on Indigenous Peoples. It is clear that even while the pandemic raged across Indigenous lands, creating what can only be considered a national crisis, coverage across national news media sources about the pandemic's impact on AI/ANs was lacking. This is not necessarily surprising, however, as previous research asserts that Native Americans are regularly missing in the media (Leavitt et al. 2015; Moore and Lanthorn 2017). While it is not our aim to prescribe what would constitute adequate coverage, the fact that Native Americans were more adversely affected by COVID-19 and yet were not a main focus of a majority of news sources clearly represents a problem.

Media are fundamental to bringing widespread attention to issues and in influencing policy, as will be discussed more in the following section. Without sufficient media coverage, issues are unlikely to gain public awareness. In an effort to highlight the role of media in garnering public and political attention to the devastation of the pandemic across Indigenous communities, this chapter examines *Times* coverage of the pandemic as it pertains specifically to Native American communities. We examined, in particular, the frequency of stories and the specific topics highlighted, paying close attention to whether stories reflected Indigenous resilience. While social media were an important channel through which information on COVID was disseminated throughout communities, national newspapers continue to influence the information spread, even indirectly through social media (Feezell 2018). For this reason, we selected to focus our attention on national newspapers rather than social media, though social media is an important area for future examination.

MEDIA INFORM THE ISSUES' SALIENCE

The importance of this project stems from the media agenda-setting literature that examines the role of the media in shaping the public's perceptions of marginalized groups. According to agenda-setting theory, the public's view of a topic as important is largely influenced by whether and how much media coverage the topic receives and how media frame the issue (McCombs 2005; McCombs, Shaw, and Weaver 2014). While earlier studies of agenda setting (e.g., Baumgartner and Jones 1995) illustrate how regular media coverage of an issue or topic directly influences whether the public believes an issue is important, current research suggests this relationship has grown more complex with the proliferation of social media and other online media platforms (Scheufele and Tewksbury 2007). Yet, even though this relationship is increasingly multifaceted, traditional media are still important for sparking public interest in political issues. King, Schneer, and White (2017), for example, find that Americans are more likely to engage in democratic politics when they are exposed to news media. Feezell (2018) and Weimann and Brosius (2016) illustrate that the agenda-setting effect is still important but has changed in concert with changing media types resulting from technological advancements. Essentially, these studies suggest that news media are still influential in shaping issue salience, and issues that lack media coverage are more likely to be overlooked.

The literature illustrates that Native Americans are relatively invisible across mass media (Campisteguy, Heilbronner, and Nakamura-Rybak 2018; Leavitt et al. 2015; Moore and Lanthorn 2017), and when they are represented, Indigenous voices are left out and presented in ways that reinforce problematic stereotypes (Eason, Brady, and Fryberg 2018; Fryberg et al. 2008; Murphy 1979; Weston 1996). Based on 2017 data, Native Americans represent "less than .05% of all journalists at leading newspapers and online publications" (Monet 2019). This unequal representation of Indigenous Peoples undoubtedly impacts how our national discourse is shaped and what issues are highlighted and how, on a daily basis. Further, there is a large body of research that examines media coverage of issues related to minority groups, yet research is comparatively lacking when it comes to examining news media coverage of Native Americans, particularly in the context of health-related topics. This is problematic because Native American communities have historically been more susceptible to contagious diseases than non-Indigenous communities, in part because Indigenous people are a communally oriented people among whom multigenerational living and community/family gatherings are common (Alvarez 2014; CDC 2009; CDC 2012; Heart and DeBruyn 1998; Stannard 1993; Reilley et al. 2014). The COVID-19 crisis is no exception (CDC 2022; Shiels et al. 2021). Native Americans additionally suffer from greater health disparities more broadly than other groups in the United States (IHS 2015). Even so, Native American nations continue to struggle to receive government assistance. While Turner's (2005) research suggests that perhaps agenda-setting literature cannot be applied equally to Indigenous and non-Indigenous political issues, a lack of media coverage will ensure that the public is unaware of these issues and does not perceive them as important. At the same time, Conner, Fryar, and Johnson (2017) suggest that low-information environments regarding Native American topics directly influence the policies that affect Native nations and that more education and knowledge would shape public opinion and, as a result, policies. During a crisis, when resources are already strained, this influence of the media could potentially impact the resources allocated to marginalized groups. These dynamics underscore the importance of analyzing how the media covered the pandemic on Indigenous lands and the extent to which Indigenous Peoples were covered at all.

THE MEDIA LEAVE NATIVE AMERICANS OUT

We selected the *New York Times* as our case for analysis because not only is it a generally well-respected news source but, compared to other top news sources, including the *Los Angeles Times*, *Washington Post*, Reuters, Associated Press, and others, by circulation (Agility PR Solutions 2022), the *Times* published significantly more unique-content articles addressing the pandemic and its impact on AI/ANs. Using the Google search engine and the *Times* online archives, we compiled a database of all news-based articles published by the *Times* on the pandemic and its impact on Native nations between January 1, 2020, and September 30, 2020, excluding commentary-based or opinion pieces, blog posts, interactive content, and briefings. We conducted multiple Google searches using the terms *NY-Times* and *New York Times*. Each term was combined with the following additional search terms, in separate searches: *COVID, coronavirus, pandemic, SARS, virus*, and *C19*. We scanned each article that came up to ensure its topic was specific to the pandemic or a pandemic-related effect. Only a few articles populated; however, based on preliminary research, we knew that the *Times* had published more articles on Native American topics than other major non-Indigenous media sources. Therefore, to expand our search, we conducted additional individual searches combining the abovementioned search terms in addition to *Native American, tribe, reservation*, and specific tribal names, such as Navajo, Hopi, and Apache, among others. These searches yielded eighteen unique-content *Times* articles about the effect of COVID-19 on Native American nations. To put that number into context, during May 2020, the month when the *Times* published the most articles (seven articles) specific to our topic, we found ninety-eight unique articles published that discussed the pandemic generally, including the seven articles specific to Native Americans. In May 2020, Native Americans were in the midst of some of the most challenging months of the pandemic, and yet only 7 percent of the COVID-related articles published by the *Times* covered their situation. Furthermore, the Navajo Nation was experiencing surging infection rates in comparison to non-Indigenous surrounding areas during April, May, and June 2020 (Eisenberg 2020; Lakhani 2021 February 4; Sottile and Ortiz 2020; Klar 2020; Powell 2020), rates that were roughly "three and a half times higher than those of white Americans" (Hlavinka 2020; Lively 2021, 2). Further, on May 10, 2020, Navajo Nation surpassed infections in any other U.S. state (Emerson and Montoya 2021; Klar 2020).

This underrepresentation in the media indicates that unless Americans specifically search for COVID-19's impact on tribal nations—and research suggests that they will not (Campisteguy, Heilbronner, and Nakamura-Rybak 2018)—they are unlikely to come across articles that discuss how much the pandemic devastated many Native American nations. From an agenda-setting perspective, this is problematic because it suggests that even while Native Americans continue to experience a lack of access to health care and little infrastructure investment from the federal government (clean water, electricity, internet access, road improvements, and more), the American public is unlikely to recognize this as a problem, and therefore, policy solutions will not be sought.

In our research, we also looked for expressions of resilience among Indigenous Peoples, which overall was an underrepresented concept in the reviewed articles. *Resilience* is an increasingly central term used in connection with Indigenous populations, specifically Native Americans and the many social struggles that are present today in Native American communities. Many of these struggles, ranging from substance abuse to physical and mental health challenges, have been recognized across disciplines as linked to colonialism and the continuing impacts of removal from land, culture, language, traditions, and so much more. There are different lenses through which we have viewed resilience over time, one being a Western colonizer lens, another an Indigenous lens. From the Western colonizer lens, resilience looks like survival during adversity, the ability to continue to exist despite some five hundred years of removal, marginalization, assimilation, warfare, and "social injustices they have experienced [beginning] with first European contact and [continuing] with postcolonial political, legal, economic, and social inequities today" (Goodkind et al. 2012, 1). It also paints a picture of victimhood and dependency.

However, from an Indigenous perspective, *resilience* means more than just survival: it describes the ability to continue to function as a society despite the continued attacks on said societal cohesion; the preservation and reinvigoration of language, cultural practices, and traditions; and the thriving of Indigenous youth and growth of Indigenous populations, despite constant attacks on their very identities. Last but not least, in the eye of crisis, whether climate change or the COVID-19 pandemic, Indigenous Peoples demonstrate resilience in their ability to adapt to swiftly changing circumstances, to lean on community and tribal government to take care of each other, and to draw from centuries of Indigenous knowledge in the approach to survival. Gerald Vizenor termed this Indigenous resilience *survivance*, which "highlight[s] Native people's individual and collective abilities to persist despite the enormous adversity imposed by colonialism. Survivance emphasizes the active presence and dynamic agency of Native peoples, in contrast to the current colonial lens of viewing American Indians in terms of absence, victimization, and powerlessness" (Goodkind et al. 2012, 2; see also Vizenor 1999). This differentiation between resilience from the colonizer lens and resilience or survivance from the Indigenous lens is important to recognize, as the former suggests victimhood and victim-based identities. The latter, however, recognizes the precontact societies, identities, practices, and more, which *continue* despite the often successful genocidal campaigns that were leveraged against America's Indigenous populations (Kroeber 2008). When we use *resilience* in our work here, we are highlighting both the colonizer lens of survival and victimhood and the Indigenous lens of continuity and *survivance*.

ARTICLE FRAMES OF THE PANDEMIC ACROSS TRIBAL LANDS

Conducting a *summative content analysis* (Hsieh and Shannon 2005) of all eighteen *Times* articles, we identified and outlined five frames through which the media might focus, to classify how each of the articles covered the issue: COVID spread, government assistance, cultural education, marginalization, and resilience.[2] For example, some articles focus on how the pandemic was spreading rapidly across tribal communities (i.e., "COVID spread"), whereas other articles highlighted how the pandemic heightened the marginalization of Indigenous groups (i.e., "marginalization"). Within each *frame*, there might be multiple *themes*. For instance, the frame "government assistance" could capture the need for government support *or* it could speak to actions on behalf of the government—two distinct themes. When sorting the eighteen *Times* articles according to overarching themes, it became apparent that two content areas dominated the publications—government assistance and cultural education—and our discussion will center on these frames. It is important to note that though we discuss the content of these two areas separately, there is much

---

2. There are a number of important limitations to this research, including the fallibility of internet searches and the algorithms that influence them. Human fallibility and bias are also important limitations, which influence the internet searches and the content analysis as a whole.

overlap, making these distinctions somewhat artificial. All but one of the eighteen articles touched on the frame of "government assistance" to some degree, and all but two articles had some element of "cultural education."

EXAMINING THE FRAME OF GOVERNMENT ASSISTANCE

The articles that touched on frames of government assistance utilized words such as *ventilator, hospital beds,* and *personal protective equipment shortages.* These terms represented government assistance vis-à-vis the extraordinary support needed to aid communities through the COVID-19 pandemic. While these discussions usually revolved around shortages, they also spoke to the U.S. federal government's attempt to supply critical health-care materials through ramped-up production, the Defense Production Act, and international purchasing. This conversation was not unique to Indigenous nations, as it has been well documented that all communities struggled to get access to basic medical supplies during the early months of the pandemic. However, Indigenous nations, which prior to the pandemic were widely known as experiencing some of the most impoverished conditions in the country, were hit particularly hard as a result of these shortages. Articles within this frame also focused on lack of access to basic resources, such as clean water and health care, highlighting a long history of need and neglect the seriousness of the conditions across Native nations. Cochrane and Walker (2020b), for example, referred to Native American nations as "critically underfunded" and "among the nation's most vulnerable communities." The Reclaiming Native Truth project found that many Americans "do not think about Native American issues," and the "lack of visibility and relevance in modern culture dehumanizes Native peoples and erodes support for Native issues." However, they also found "that when people are exposed to accurate facts about Native American history and contemporary life, they believe the information, feel cheated that they didn't learn it in school, and quickly become more open to a new narrative" (Campisteguy, Heilbronner, and Nakamura-Rybak 2018, 8). It is reasonable to argue, then, that this reporting by the *Times* could have helped bring attention to Native Americans' challenges around COVID-19 and spark more political support and social pressure—at least among those who read the *Times.*

Also widely discussed in many of the articles were federal stimulus payments, the role of Alaska Native Corporations, and the juggling of tribal needs and constituents. Most Americans do not have a clear (or any) understanding of the ways in which federal Indian policy stipulates government-to-government relations with Indigenous nations. This complicates not just the understanding among non-Native citizens of how sovereign Indigenous nations intersect with state governments and local municipalities, but it also impacts non-Native policymakers, government officials, first responders, and law enforcement agencies that act around and on tribal lands. States and federally recognized tribes are both subjects under federal law, and neither have jurisdiction over one another. In 2022, there were 574 federally recognized tribes in the United States, including 229 nations in Alaska, each of which is considered a sovereign but domestic dependent nation (Bens 2020; Gordon 2018). Some of the Alaska Native tribes are organized as so-called Alaska Native Corporations, whose receipt of CARES Act funding in 2020 sparked controversy. This controversy culminated in *Yellen v. Confederated Tribes of the Chehalis Reservation* (2021), in which the U.S. Supreme Court ruled that Alaska Native Corporations are equal in status to federally recognized tribes and eligible to receive federal funding (Gresko 2021). This decision is understood as a possible challenge to tribal sovereignty and the role of federally recognized tribes, according to former Navajo Nation president Jonathan Nez (Gresko 2021).

Clearly, the relationship between Alaskan Native Corporations, federally recognized tribes, and the federal government is complex. Yet, *Times* articles do not provide much background when discussing the legal challenges that arose. A couple of the stories do discuss the for-profit nature of Alaskan Native Corporations and provide surface-level context to the disputes (e.g., Cochrane and Walker 2020a; Cochrane and Walker 2020b; Walker and Cochrane 2020a), while one article (Romero 2020c) mentions the legal situation but does not provide any explanation or background. Also important to mention, though beyond the scope of this particular project, Cochrane and Walker's (2020b) use of the word *battle* to describe the legal disputes between Native nations and the Alaskan Native Corporations seems to reinforce the militant or factionalism frames identified in the media by Baylor (1996), even while providing some of the most in-depth educational background to the dispute.

Times articles in our analysis do discuss delay in or halting of the disbursement of CARES Act funds and mounting pressure for Indigenous nations to sue the federal government over the already allocated funding (e.g., Cochrane and Walker 2020b). The reviewed articles additionally feature discussion of stimulus payments and how they would affect tribal populations. One of the *Times* articles, for instance, suggests that the stimulus amounts do not reflect accurate tribal enrollments, as the U.S. Department of the Treasury is alleged to have used U.S. Department of Housing and Urban Development (HUD) data, which is based on "how many people within a certain geographic area identif[y] as American Indian or Alaska Native on their census forms" (Cochrane and Walker 2020b). HUD's approach to eligibility does not consider how tribal enrollment functions from nation to nation or which Indigenous nations experienced termination in the 1950s. In addition, nations without designated reservation land or territory returned populations of zero, meaning thousands of enrolled members were excluded from stimulus accounting. Historically, Native nations have struggled with enrollment numbers. Many tribal communities were weakened by federal efforts encouraging Indigenous people to leave their ancestral lands and move into cities, effectively giving up their tribal affiliations (i.e., the Voluntary Relocation Program), or were stripped of their trust relationship with the U.S. government and their ancestral land sold off to private ownership (Wilkins 2016). Much of this was driven by the termination policies of the 1950s, when some 109 Native nations were stripped of their federal recognition and over 12,500 Indigenous people were relocated to cities. Many others moved to the cities for vocational training, college education, and, subsequently, employment opportunities (Ulrich 2010; Wilkins 2016). These are significant reasons for why roughly 80 percent of Native Americans do not live on reservations (Leggat-Barr, Uchikoshi, and Goldman 2021), with varying numbers living in cities and border towns across the nation. Overall, the number of "urban Indians" in cities today has grown from about 8 percent in the 1950s to 64 percent in 2000 (National Archives 2023), and early reports of the 2020 census suggest an increase in the overall Indigenous population to 86.5 percent (*Indian Country Today* 2021). For many urban Indigenous people, this means loss of some or all connection to their Indigenous heritage; for others, it means simultaneously living in two worlds. Ultimately, the termination efforts were unsuccessful, and most nations were able to retain or regain federal recognition and preserve the trust relationship, highlighting sur-vivance—or the resilience of America's first people. These themes were touched upon in the *Times* articles, yet neither survivance nor resilience were explicitly identified or central to most of the stories.

EXAMINING THE FRAME OF CULTURAL EDUCATION

Articles that primarily touched on themes related to the "cultural education" frame grappled with challenges that arguably are products of settler colo-nialism and its long history of federal neglect of and hostility toward Indig-enous Peoples in the United States. Such challenges include today's IHS, which has struggled with funding, equipment, and accessibility for a long time (Warne and Frizzell 2014). Furthermore, notoriously limited access to running and clean water, challenges that arise from multigenerational living (CDC 2021), widespread poverty, food deserts with limited access to fresh foods, and the role of border towns in the spread of COVID-19 on the Navajo reservation were prominently featured (e.g., Krishna 2020; Romero and Healy 2020; Walker 2020a). A study on COVID risk fac-tors and mortality notes that the Navajo Nation, "[which] has garnered considerable media attention due to its high rates of COVID-19 infection and mortality, has some of the highest water and plumbing insecurity in the U.S. with about 40 percent of families lacking running water in their homes" (Leggat-Barr, Uchikoshi, and Goldman 2021, 1190). This theme also highlights some discussion around resilience, as tribal government efforts to protect their people are described as drawing from Indigenous cultural practices and the implicit responsibility for those governments to distribute resources and attempt to stop the spread within their commu-nities despite challenges from state governments (e.g., South Dakota). The discussion of Alaska Native Corporations and their eligibility for stimulus funding surfaced in this theme as well. At the core of these portrayals was the definition of "tribal government," which was central to the challenge brought to the U.S. Supreme Court in *Yellen v. Confederated Tribes of the Chehalis Reservation.* This coverage, while lacking in detail, brought to public attention the complicated legal boundaries and intergovernmental relationships that define interactions between the federal government and Native nations. These stories also highlight that the federal government has leeway in recognizing Indigenous nations/peoples based on selective use of statistics and how representative bodies are defined.

Some articles focused on mitigation efforts of the tribal governments, for example the Navajo Nation curfew orders. The curfews effectively locked down the Navajo Nation on weekdays from evening to early morning for several months (Hay 2020). Later in the pandemic, this also included weekend lockdowns. There is discussion on how earlier on in the pandemic, the National Guard was involved in setting up a field hospital on the Navajo Nation, along with providing other services, including distributing personal protective equipment (e.g., Romero 2020a). Additional article topics included anti–Native American racism, where people blamed Navajo for "bringing" COVID-19 to border towns (Romero 2020a, 2020c; Walker 2020a); sovereignty (Romero and Healy 2020; Walker and Cochrane 2020b); Native American businesses and casinos in California (Fuller 2020; Krishna 2020; Romero and Healy 2020); Native nations' lack of proximity to medical care (Yan 2020); European conquest and a history of diseases such as smallpox, bubonic plague, typhus, influenza (1918 pandemic), and hantavirus (1993 outbreak) (Krishna 2020; Romero 2020a); the Trail of Tears (O'Loughlin and Zaveri 2020); impacts on economic pursuits (Brown 2020; Romero and Healy 2020); Indigenous cultural activities, family structure and clans, matriarchy, and kinship systems (*ké*) (Brown 2020; Krishna 2020); the Long Walk of 1864 (Nierenberg 2020); and treaties and federal policies (Walker and Cochrane 2020b). Some of these articles went more in-depth than others in educating readers on the background of Indigenous, and more specifically Navajo, cultures. In summary, reporting on the catastrophic spread of COVID-19 on the Navajo reservation opened a window for nationwide readership into Indigenous lives, challenges, and practices, and emphasized a need for political leadership to address colonial history that has systematically marginalized, ostracized, and neglected the original inhabitants of this country.

EXAMINING THE FRAME OF RESILIENCE

Overall, about half of the articles mentioned topics related to resilience, but often in just a sentence or two about the ways in which tribal governments were combating the pandemic and its impacts. Five articles specifically highlighted how Indigenous Peoples were drawing from their cultural heritage to address COVID-related problems. For instance, one journalist stated that "[the] Oglala Sioux, like many other Native Americans across the country, are relying on the practices—seed saving, canning, dehydrating—that their forebears developed to survive harsh conditions, with limited supplies" (Krishna 2020). While none of the articles highlighted resilience or survivance as a topic generally, or specifically emphasized the strength of Indigenous Peoples to mitigate problems, this sentence illustrated an example of such resilience. Many of the articles were written by Indigenous journalists or provide quotes from tribal members and, as such, emphasize practices using Indigenous knowledge and traditional ways of survival, which highlight nothing less than Indigenous resilience in the face of yet another crisis. However, the *Times* articles still reflect some of the language of conquest and stereotypes, failing to outright name the resilience that Indigenous people have shown in the face of colonization and continued crises and challenges to survival. These themes can be found and picked out by the knowing reader, but they are not at the core of the already scant reporting. For instance, Indigenous Peoples have relied heavily on their tribal governments to procure federal aid, to distribute food and resource assistance locally, and to pass regulations that would stop the spread of COVID-19 and ultimately keep tribal members safe. These topics show up in the reporting in the form of the clashes that many of these regulations created with nontribal jurisdictions, which mostly centered on lockdowns and curfews prohibiting interstate commerce, tourism, and other travel across sovereign Indigenous land, which created further challenges on the jurisdictional level, in regard to state highways, federal trust land, and Indigenous governance (e.g., the conflict with Governor Noem in South Dakota). None of the *Times* articles, nor those distributed by the Associated Press or Reuters, reported on the positive interventions, such as dramatically reducing the spread among tribal members with rigorous contact tracing (e.g., the White Mountain Apache Tribe; see Kolata 2020), or the immense successes that many Indigenous tribes recorded in keeping death tolls down (e.g., the Cheyenne River Sioux Tribe). Instead, the primary focus was on the Navajo Nation—which spans the largest geographical area across three states and seven counties and has the largest Indigenous population living on tribal land—and its fight to keep the virus from spreading among their often remote communities. These major news outlets paid little attention to the incredible level of survivance demonstrated by people without access to running, or even uncontaminated, water; the strength of the Navajo people to care for their elders, families, livestock, and land, despite long distances on remote dirt roads; and the exemplary governance demonstrated by the Jonathan Nez and Myron Lizer administration.

CONCLUSIONS

It is important to recognize that media coverage of the pandemic across Native American communities has been largely inadequate. Native Americans are among the groups most impacted by the pandemic, and yet their stories have been relatively ignored across the national media. The *Times* covered the issue more robustly than any of the other top ten news outlets that we reviewed, and yet still only published eighteen news-based articles over the course of nine months on the issue of Native Americans and the pandemic. This is in comparison to ninety-eight articles on the pandemic generally in May 2020 alone—only 7 percent of which touch on Native American topics. Further, a generic Google search for *Times* articles on the pandemic broadly did not populate articles on Native Americans. This is telling in itself, and worth further investigation. Our findings indicate that unless people are specifically searching for the pandemic's impact on Native nations, they are unlikely to come across articles that discuss how it impacted them.

The lack of media coverage is problematic because, according to agenda-setting theory, lack of media coverage contributes to limited (if any) public awareness of an issue, perpetuating a lack of interest among the public on Native American topics. While our methods do not allow us to determine here whether greater media coverage would have garnered enough public interest to pressure the national government into better supporting AI/ANs during the most challenging months of the pandemic, agenda-setting theory would suggest that greater media attention likely could have pressured the U.S. government to adopt policy solutions that would have provided greater support to Native nations and earlier on in the pandemic. Further complicating this hypothesis is the fact the Trump administration was notoriously "at war" with the national media. This makes it even less clear to what extent more media coverage would have mitigated some of the challenges AI/ANs had to endure just to receive federal support.

We find, however, that the *Times* articles do reflect on the social inequities that settler colonialism and federal Indian law have fostered in the past five centuries, even though in many cases this background is only minimally discussed. Native American nations have shown resilience in the face of extermination, relocation, marginalization, broken treaties and promises, and more. The absence of reporting on Indigenous Peoples in the United States, as we highlighted in this chapter, is representative of a general nationwide neglect of Indigenous societies. This neglect appears to have become even more apparent during such a major event as the COVID-19 pandemic. Yet the *Times* has managed to capture what we termed "cultural education," which was prevalent across the majority of the analyzed newspaper articles, and does also highlight elements of resilience, though this is limited. Each of these articles provides snippets of information and background on Indigenous realities in the United States. As a result, this coverage on behalf of the *Times* might be a first step toward bringing greater attention to Indigenous topics, as called for by the Reclaiming Native Truth report (Campisteguy, Heilbronner, and Nakamura-Rybak 2018).

It is important to note that the *Times* has been criticized for its bias and use of clichés about Native Americans (Native American Journalists Association 2021), and research suggests that even "objective" news stories frequently promote stereotypical frames about Native Americans (Miller and Ross 2004). Miller and Ross further argue that "objective" news stories perpetuate representations of Native Americans as "degraded outsiders," which "may inhibit the ability of American Indians to act effectively or be taken seriously by readers in context related to significant issues, such as tribal sovereignty and culture" (2004, 255). However, the aim of this chapter is not to identify whether the *Times* coverage uses these stereotypes in their reporting, since research already suggests they do, but rather whether it published stories around topics that are important to a general understanding of the scope of the challenges faced by Native Americans. Yet it is important to recognize that how articles are framed can contribute to negative public perceptions and can reinforce problematic stereotypes (Eason, Brady, and Fryberg 2018; Conner, Fryar, and Johnson 2017; Fryberg et al. 2008; McQuail 1994; Murphy 1979; Weston

1996). Therefore, a more detailed analysis of the wording of the published articles and the particular stereotypical frames they might perpetuate is important for future research.

REFERENCES

Abou-Sabe, Kenzi, Cynthia McFadden, Christine Romo, and Jaime Longoria. 2020. "Coronavirus Batters the Navajo Nation, and It's About to Get Worse." *NBC News*, April 20, 2020. https://www.nbcnews.com/health/health-news /coronavirus-batters-navajo-nation-it-s-about-get-worse-n1187501.

Agility PR Solutions. 2022. "Top 10 U.S. Newspapers by Circulation." Last updated July 2022. https://www.agilitypr.com/resources/top-media-outlets/top -10-daily-american-newspapers/.

Alvarez, Alex. 2014. *Native America and the Question of Genocide*. Lanham, MD: Rowman & Littlefield.

Associated Press. "Navajo President: Tribe Can't Afford a Large COVID-19 Surge." December 10, 2021. https://apnews.com/article/coronavirus-pandemic -business-lifestyle-health-arizona-7f7ca1732bb612c1dbf9b7cd3aa0a378.

Baumgartner, Frank, and Bryan D. Jones. 1995. *Agendas and Instability in American Politics*. Chicago: University of Chicago Press.

Baylor, Tim. 1996. "Media Framing of Movement Protest: The Case of American Indian Protest." *Social Science Journal* 33, no. 3: 241–56. https://doi.org/10.1016 /S0362-3319(96)90021-X.

Beitsch, Rebecca. 2020. "Judge Orders Mnuchin to Give Native American Tribes Full Stimulus Funding." *The Hill*, June 17, 2020. https://thehill.com/policy /energy-environment/503175-judge-orders-mnuchin-to-give-tribes-full-stim ulus-funding.

Bens, Jonas. 2020. "'Domestic Dependent Nations' and Indigenous Identity: *Cherokee Nation v. Georgia*." In *The Indigenous Paradox*, 51–69. Philadelphia: University of Pennsylvania Press.

Bowing, Joshua. 2020. "Surprise Mayor Hall Announces He's Tested Positive for COVID-19." *Arizona Republic*, June 18, 2020. https://azcentral.newspapers .com/image/668451177/?terms=ducey%20%2B%20mask&match=1.

Brown, Patricia L. 2020. "On Tribal Lands, Time to Make Art for Solace and Survival." *New York Times*, June 19, 2020. https://www.nytimes.com/2020/06/05 /arts/design/native-americans-art-coronavirus.html?searchResultPosition=8.

Burki, Talha. 2021. "COVID-19 Among American Indians and Alaska Natives." *Lancet Infectious Diseases* 21, no. 3: 325–26. https://doi.org/10.1016/S1473-3099 (21)00083-9.

Campisteguy, Maria E., Jennifer M. Heilbronner, and Corinne Nakamura-Rybak. 2018. *Reclaiming Native Truth: Research Findings; Compilation of All Research*. Longmont, CO: First Nations Development Institute and Echo Hawk Consulting. https://www.firstnations.org/wp-content/uploads/2018/12/Full FindingsReport-screen.pdf.

Cancryn, Adam. 2020. "Exclusive: Emergency Coronavirus Funds for American Indian Health Stalled." *Politico*, March 20, 2020. https://www.politico.com /news/2020/03/20/coronavirus-american-indian-health-138724.

CDC (Centers for Disease Control and Prevention). 2009. "Deaths Related to 2009 Pandemic Influenza A (H1N1) Among American Indian/Alaska Natives—12 States, 2009." *Morbidity Mortality Weekly Report* 58, no. 48: 1341–44. https://www.ncbi.nlm.nih.gov/pubmed/20010508.

CDC (Centers for Disease Control and Prevention). 2012. *Sexually Transmitted Disease Surveillance 2011*. Atlanta: U.S. Department of Health and Human Services, December 2012. https://www.cdc.gov/std/stats/archive/Surv2011.pdf.

CDC (Centers for Disease Control and Prevention). 2021. "Guidance and Tips for Tribal Community Living During COVID-19." Last updated August 23, 2022. https://www.cdc.gov/coronavirus/2019-ncov/community/tribal/social -distancing.html.

CDC (Centers for Disease Control and Prevention). 2022. "Hospitalization and Death by Race/Ethnicity." Last updated May 25, 2023. https://www.cdc.gov /coronavirus/2019-ncov/covid-data/investigations-discovery/hospitalization -death-by-race-ethnicity.html#footnote03.

Cochrane, Emily, and Mark Walker. 2020a. "Federal Watchdog to Examine Official's Role in Tribal Fund Distribution." *New York Times*, May 11, 2020. https:// www.nytimes.com/2020/05/11/us/politics/native-american-tribes-corona virus-funds.html?searchResultPosition=12.

Cochrane, Emily, and Mark Walker. 2020b. "Tribes in a Battle for Their Share of Virus Stimulus Money." *New York Times*, June 19, 2020. https://www.nytimes .com/2020/06/19/us/politics/tribes-coronavirus-stimulus.html?searchResult Position=10.

Conner, Thaddieus, Alisa H. Fryar, and Tyler Johnson. 2017. "Information Versus Ideology: Shaping Attitudes Towards Native American Policy." *Social Science Journal* 54, no. 1: 56–66. https://doi.org/10.1016/j.soscij.2016.11.001.

CRC (Johns Hopkins University and Medicine Coronavirus Resource Center). n.d. "COVID-19 Dashboard." Accessed December 3, 2021. https://corona virus.jhu.edu/map.html.

Deloria, Philip S. 1986. "The Era of Indian Self-Determination: An Overview." In *Indian Self-Rule: First-Hand Accounts of Indian-White Relations from Roosevelt to Reagan*, edited by Kenneth R. Philp, 191–94. Denver: University Press of Colorado.

Deloria, Vine, Jr. 2010. *Behind the Trail of Broken Treaties: An Indian Declaration of Independence*. Austin: University of Texas Press.

Diethelm, Lisa. 2020. "Tribes Say Delayed Coronavirus Funds Hurt Relief, Other Efforts." *Cronkite News*, July 11, 2020, https://ktar.com/story/3381289/tribes-say-delayed-coronavirus-funds-hurt-relief-other-efforts/.

Eason, Arianne E., Laura M. Brady, and Stephanie A. Fryberg. 2018. "Reclaiming Representations and Interrupting the Cycle of Bias against Native Americans." *Daedalus* 147, no. 2 (Spring): 70–81. https://doi.org/10.1162/DAED_a_00491.

Eisenberg, Kate. 2020. "Updating COVID-19 Data for Navajo Counties." *Kate Eisenberg MD* (blog), April 7, 2020. https://www.kateeisenbergmd.com/blog/updating-covid-19-for-navajo-counties.

Emerson, Marc A., and Teresa Montoya. 2021 "Confronting Legacies of Structural Racism and Settler Colonialism to Understand COVID-19 Impacts on the Navajo Nation." *American Journal of Public Health* 111, no. 8 (August): 1465–69. https://doi.org/10.2105/ajph.2021.306398.

Feezell, Jessica T. 2018. "Agenda Setting Through Social Media: The Importance of Incidental News Exposure and Social Filtering in the Digital Era." *Political Research Quarterly* 71, no. 2: 482–94. https://doi.org/10.1177/1065912917744895.

Fonseca, Felicia. 2020. "Judge: U.S. Must Release $679M in Tribal Virus Relief Funds." Associated Press, June 15, 2020. https://apnews.com/article/us-news-health-courts-sd-state-wire-virus-outbreak-e8869b31e0d9b35dfe5d00393ddf67f6.

Fryberg, Stephanie. A., Hazel Rose Markus, Daphna Oyserman, and Joseph M. Stone. 2008. "Of Warrior Chiefs and Indian Princesses: The Psychological Consequences of American Indian Mascots." *Basic and Applied Social Psychology* 30, no. 3: 208–18. https://doi.org/10.1080/01973530802375003.

Fuller, Thomas. 2020. "Asserting Sovereignty, Indian Casinos Defy California's Governor and Reopen." *New York Times*, May 28, 2020. https://www.nytimes.com/2020/05/28/us/california-virus-casinos.html?searchResultPosition=10.

Goodkind, Jessica R., Julia M. Hess, Beverly Gorman, and Danielle P. Parker. 2012. "'We're Still in a Struggle': Diné Resilience, Survival, Historical Trauma, and Healing." *Qualitative Health Research* 22, no. 8: 1019–36. https://doi.org/10.1177/1049732312450324.

Gordon, Theodor P. 2018. *Cahuilla Nation Activism and the Tribal Casino Movement*. Reno: University of Nevada Press.

Gresko, Jessica. "Supreme Court Sides with Alaska Natives in COVID-19 Aid Case." Associated Press, June 25, 2021, https://apnews.com/article/us-supreme

-court-alaska-health-coronavirus-pandemic-business-8107f2e49fdc150af7cf0c
fcdc2f449c.

Hay, Andrew. 2020. "Facing Arizona Surge, Navajos Reimpose Virus Curfew."
Reuters, June 17, 2020. https://www.reuters.com/article/us-health-coronavirus
-usa-navajo/facing-arizona-surge-navajos-reimpose-virus-curfew-idUSKBN
23O3R4.

Heart, Maria Y. H. B., and Lemyra M. DeBruyn.1998. "The American Indian
Holocaust: Healing Historical Unresolved Grief." *American Indian and Alaska
Native Mental Health Research* 8, no. 2: 56–78. https://pubmed.ncbi.nlm.nih
.gov/9842066/.

Hlavinka, Elizabeth. 2020. "CDC Confirms Soaring COVID-19 Rate Among
Native Americans." *MedPage Today*, August 19, 2020. https://www.medpage
today.com/infectiousdisease/covid19/88167#:~:text=CDC%20Confirms
%20Soaring%20COVID%2D19%20Rate%20Among%20Native%20
Americans.

Hsieh, Hsiu-Fang, and Sarah E. Shannon. 2005. "Three Approaches to Qualitative Content Analysis." *Qualitative Health. Research* 15, no. 9: 1277–88. https://
doi.org/10.1177/1049732305276687.

IHS (Indian Health Service). 2015. *Trends in Indian Health: 2014 Edition*. Rockville, MD: Indian Health Service, Division of Program Statistics, March 2015.
https://www.ihs.gov/sites/dps/themes/responsive2017/display_objects/docu
ments/Trends2014Book508.pdf.

IHS (Indian Health Service). 2023. "Coronavirus (COVID-19)." Last updated
June 29, 2023. https://www.ihs.gov/coronavirus/?CFID=36476569&CF
TOKEN=55883207.

Indian Country Today. 2021. "2020 Census: Native Population Increased by 86.5
Percent." August 13, 2021. https://indiancountrytoday.com/news/2020-census
-native-population-increased-by-86-5-percent.

Innes, Stephanie. 2020. "Report: COVID-19 Policies Effective." *Arizona Republic*,
October 12, 2020. https://azcentral.newspapers.com/image/687622122/?terms
=ducey%20%2B%20mask&match=1.

Jewell, Sally. 2014. "Reaffirmation of the Federal Trust Responsibility to Federally
Recognized Indian Tribes and Individual Indian Beneficiaries." August 20,
2014. https://www.doi.gov/sites/doi.gov/files/migrated/news/pressreleases
/upload/Signed-SO-3335.pdf.

Joe, Mariella. 2020. "A Plea from the Navajo Nation, Written by Nina Ritchie,
M.D., MedPeds Physician." Facebook, April 2, 2020. https://www.facebook
.com/mari.joe.98/posts/pfbid0DmjM3vuqE1JqD29Q8wWZj5aw28VQEK
NYt4SM9FWBbj6Ph7DuiQmYqYAwQAobTRe3l.

Jones, David S. 2006. "The Persistence of American Indian Health Disparities." *American Journal of Public Health* 96: 2122–34. https://doi.org/10.2105
%2FAJPH.2004.054262.

King, Gary, Benjamin Schneer, and Ariel White. 2017. "How the News Media
Activate Public Expression and Influence National Agendas." *Science* 358,
no. 6364: 776–80. https://doi.org/10.1126/science.aao1100.

Klar, Rebecca. 2020. "Navajo Nation Reports More Coronavirus Cases Per Capita
than Any US State." *The Hill*, May 11, 2020. https://thehill.com/policy/health
care/497091-navajo-nation-has-more-coronavirus-cases-per-capita-than-any
-us-state.

Klemko, Robert. 2020. "Coronavirus Has Been Devastating to the Navajo Nation,
and Help for a Complex Fight Has Been Slow." *Washington Post*, May 11,
2020. https://www.washingtonpost.com/national/coronavirus-navajo-nation
-crisis/2020/05/11/b2a35c4e-91fe-11ea-a0bc-4e9ad4866d21_story.html.

Kolata, Gina. 2020. "On Native American Land, Contact Tracing Is Saving Lives."
New York Times, August 13, 2020. https://www.nytimes.com/2020/08/13/health
/coronavirus-contact-tracing-apaches.html?searchResultPosition=3.

Krishna, Priya. 2020. "How Native Americans Are Fighting a Food Crisis." *New
York Times*, April 13, 2020. https://www.nytimes.com/2020/04/13/dining/native
-americans-coronavirus.html?searchResultPosition=20.

Kroeber, Karl. 2008. "Why It's a Good Thing Gerald Vizenor Is Not an Indian."
In *Survivance: Narratives of Native Presence*, edited by Gerald Vizenor, 25–38.
Lincoln: University of Nebraska Press.

Lakhani, Nina. 2020a. "Native American Tribe Takes Trailblazing Steps to Fight
Covid-19 Outbreak." *The Guardian*, March 18, 2020. https://www.theguardian
.com/us-news/2020/mar/18/covidcoronavirus-native-american-lummi-nation
-trailblazing-steps.

Lakhani, Nina. 2020b. "Navajo Nation Reels Under Weight of Coronavirus—and
History of Broken Promises." *The Guardian*, May 8, 2020. https://www.the
guardian.com/world/2020/may/08/navajo-nation-coronavirus.

Lakhani, Nina. 2021. "Exclusive: Indigenous Americans Dying from Covid at
Twice the Rate of White Americans." *The Guardian*, February 4, 2021, https://
www.theguardian.com/us-news/2021/feb/04/native-americans-coronavirus
-covid-death-rate.

Leavitt, Peter A., Rebecca Covarrubias, Yvonne A. Perez, and Stephanie A. Fryberg. 2015. "'Frozen in Time': The Impact of Native American Media Representations on Identity and Self-Understanding." *Journal of Social Issues* 71,
no. 1: 39–53. https://doi.org/10.1111/josi.12095.

Leggat-Barr, Katherine, Fumiya Uchikoshi, and Noreen Goldman. 2021. "COVID-19 Risk Factors and Mortality Among Native Americans." *Demographic Research* 45: 1185–1218. https://dx.doi.org/10.4054/DemRes.2021.45.39.

Lively, Cathy P. 2021. "COVID-19 in the Navajo Nation Without Access to Running Water: The Lasting Effects of Settler Colonialism." *Voices in Bioethics* 7. https://doi.org/10.7916/vib.v7i.7889.

Martinez, Ramon, III. 2022. "COVID-19 and the Missouri Workforce." MOST Policy Initiative, February 8, 2022. https://mostpolicyinitiative.org/wp-content/uploads/2022/02/COVID-19-and-the-Missouri-Workforce.pdf.

McCombs, Maxwell. 2005. "A Look at Agenda Setting: Past, Present and Future." *Journalism Studies* 6, no. 4: 543–57. https://doi.org/10.1080/14616700500250438.

McCombs, Maxwell E., Donald L. Shaw, and David H. Weaver. 2014. "New Directions in Agenda-Setting Theory and Research." *Mass Communication and Society* 17, no. 6: 781–802. https://doi.org/10.1080/15205436.2014.964871.

McQuail, Dennis. 1994. *Mass Communication Theory: An Introduction*. 2nd ed. Thousand Oaks, CA: Sage Publishing.

Miller, Autumn, and Susan Dente Ross. 2004. "They Are Not Us: Framing of American Indians by the *Boston Globe*." *Harvard Journal of Communications* 15: 245–59. https://doi.org/10.1177/0196859914537304.

Monet, Jenni. 2019. "The Crisis in Covering Indian Country." *Columbia Journalism Review*, March 29, 2019. https://www.cjr.org/opinion/Indigenous-journalism-erasure.php.

Moore, Ellen E., and Kylie R. Lanthorn. 2017. "Framing Disaster: News Media Coverage of Environmental Justice." *SIAS Faculty Publications* 782. https://digitalcommons.tacoma.uw.edu/ias_pub/782.

Murphy, Sharon. 1979. "American Indians and the Media: Neglect and Stereotype." *Journalism History* 6, no. 2: 39–43. https://doi.org/10.1080/00947679.1979.12066911.

National Archives. 2023. "American Indian Urban Relocation." Lasted updated March 3, 2023. https://www.archives.gov/education/lessons/indian-relocation.html.

Native American Journalists Association. 2021. "2021 NAJA Media Spotlight Report." https://najanewsroom.com/2021-naja-media-spotlight-report/.

NCAI (National Congress of American Indians). 2020. *Tribal Nations and the United States: An Introduction*. Washington, D.C.: National Congress of American Indians, February 2020. http://www.ncai.org/tribalnations/introduction/Tribal_Nations_and_the_United_States_An_Introduction-web-.pdf.

NDOH (Navajo Department of Health). 2023. "Dikos Ntsaaígíí-19 (COVID-19)." Last updated May 4, 2023. https://www.ndoh.navajo-nsn.gov/covid-19.

NIHB (National Indian Health Board). n.d. "COVID-19 Tribal Resource Center." Accessed October 20, 2021. https://www.nihb.org/covid-19/.

Nierenberg, Amelia. 2020. "For the Navajo Nation, a Fight for Better Food Gains New Urgency." *New York Times*, August 3, 2020. https://www.nytimes.com/2020/08/03/dining/navajo-nation-food-coronavirus.html?searchResult Position=5.

O'Brien, Brendan. 2020. "South Dakota Governor Threatens Tribes with Legal Action on Checkpoints." Reuters, May 11, 2020. https://www.reuters.com/article/health-coronavirus-usa-checkpoints/south-dakota-governor-threatens-tribes-with-legal-action-on-checkpoints-idUSKBN22N30U.

O'Loughlin, Ed, and Mihir Zaveri. 2020. "Irish Return an Old Favor, Helping Native Americans Battling the Virus." *New York Times*, May 5, 2020. https://www.nytimes.com/2020/05/05/world/coronavirus-ireland-native-american-tribes.html?searchResultPosition=13.

Ortiz, Erik. 2020. "Native American Health Center Asked for COVID-19 Supplies. It Got Body Bags Instead." *NBC News*, May 5, 2020. https://www.nbcnews.com/news/us-news/native-american-health-center-asked-covid-19-supplies-they-got-n1200246.

Powell, Kim. 2020. "Navajo Nation Continues Strict Curfews Due to 'Uncontrolled Spread' of COVID-19." *Arizona's Family*, December 28, 2020. https://perma.cc/GTF2-9JU6.

Power, Tamara, Denise Wilson, Odette Best, Teresa Brockie, Lisa Bourque Bearskin, Eugenia Millender, and John Lowe. 2020. "COVID-19 and Indigenous Peoples: An Imperative for Action." *Journal of Clinical Nursing* 29, no. 15–16: 2737–41. https://doi.org/10.1111/jocn.15320.

Qeadan, Fares, Elizabeth VanSant-Webb, Benjamin Tingey, Tiana N. Rogers, Ellen Brooks, Nana A. Mensah, Karen M. Winkfield, Ali I. Saeed, Kevin English, and Charles R. Rogers. 2021. "Racial Disparities in COVID-19 Outcomes Exist Despite Comparable Elixhauser Comorbidity Indices Between Blacks, Hispanics, Native Americans, and Whites." *Scientific Reports* 11, no. 1: 1–11. https://doi.org/10.1038/s41598-021-88308-2.

Reilley, Brigg, Emily Bloss, Kathy K. Byrd, Jonathan Iralu, Lisa Neel, and James Cheek. 2014. "Death Rates from Human Immunodeficiency Virus and Tuberculosis Among American Indians/Alaska Natives in the United States, 1990–2009." *American Journal of Public Health* 104, no. S3: S453–59. https://doi.org/10.2105%2FAJPH.2013.301746.

Rodriguez-Lonebear, Desi, Nicolás E. Barceló, Randall Akee, and Stephanie Russo Carroll. 2020. "American Indian Reservations and COVID-19: Correlates of Early Infection Rates in the Pandemic." *Journal of Public Health Management and Practice* 26, no. 4: 371–77. https://doi.org/10.1097/phh.000 0000000001206.

Romero, Simon. 2020a. "Checkpoints, Curfews, Airlifts: Virus Rips through Navajo Nation." *New York Times*, April 9, 2020. https://www.nytimes.com/2020 /04/09/us/coronavirus-navajo-nation.html?searchResultPosition=22.

Romero, Simon. 2020b. "How New Mexico, One of the Poorest States, Averted a Steep Death Toll." *New York Times*, April 24, 2020. https://www.nytimes .com/2020/04/24/us/coronavirus-new-mexico.html?searchResultPosition=1.

Romero, Simon. 2020c. "New Mexico Invokes Riot Law to Control Virus near Navajo Nation." *New York Times*, May 4, 2020. https://www.nytimes.com /2020/05/04/us/coronavirus-new-mexico-gallup-navajo.html?searchResult Position=16.

Romero, Simon, and Jack Healy. 2020. "Tribal Nations Face Most Severe Crisis in Decades as the Coronavirus Closes Casinos." *New York Times*, May 11, 2020. https://www.nytimes.com/2020/05/11/us/coronavirus-native-americans -indian-country.html?searchResultPosition=14.

Scheufele, Dietram A., and David Tewksbury. 2007. "Framing, Agenda Setting, and Priming: The Evolution of Three Media Effects Models." *Journal of Communication* 57: 9–20. https://doi.org/10.1111/j.0021-9916.2007.00326.x.

Shiels, Meredith S., Anika T. Haque, Emily A. Haozous, Paul S. Albert, Jonas S. Almeida, Montserrat García-Closas, Anna M. Nápoles, Eliseo J. Pérez-Stable, Neal D. Freedman, Amy Berrington de González. 2021. "Racial and Ethnic Disparities in Excess Death During the COVID-19 Pandemic, March to December 2020." *Annals of Internal Medicine* (December). https://doi.org/10 .7326/M21-2134.

Sottile, Chiara, and Erik Ortiz. 2020. "Coronavirus Hits Indian Country Hard, Exposing Infrastructure Disparities." *NBC News*, April 19, 2020. https:// www.nbcnews.com/news/us-news/coronavirus-hits-indian-country-hard -exposing-infrastructure-disparities-n1186976.

Stannard, David, E. 1993. *American Holocaust: The Conquest of the New World*. New York: Oxford University Press.

Tai, Don Bambino Geno, Aditya Shah, Chyke A. Doubeni, Irene G. Sia, and Mark L. Wieland. 2021. "The Disproportionate Impact of COVID-19 on Racial and Ethnic Minorities in The United States." *Clinical Infectious Diseases* 72, no. 4: 703–6. https://doi.org/10.1093/cid/ciaa815.

Turner, Charles C. 2005. *The Politics of Minor Concerns: American Indian Policy and Congressional Dynamics*. Lanham, MD: University Press of America.

Ulrich, Roberta. 2010. *American Indian Nations from Termination to Restoration, 1953–2006*. Lincoln: University of Nebraska Press.

van Dorn, Aaron, Rebecca E. Cooney, and Miriam L. Sabin. 2000. "COVID-19 Exacerbating Inequalities in the US." *Lancet* 395, no. 10232: 1243–44. https://doi.org/10.1016/S0140-6736(20)30893-X.

Walker, Mark. 2020a. "Pandemic Highlights Deep-Rooted Problems in Indian Health Service." *New York Times*, September 29, 2020. https://www.nytimes.com/2020/09/29/us/politics/coronavirus-indian-health-service.html?search ResultPosition=2.

Walker, Mark. 2020b. "'A Devastating Blow': Virus Kills 81 Members of Native American Tribe." *New York Times*, October 8, 2020. https://www.nytimes.com/2020/10/08/us/choctaw-indians-coronavirus.html.

Walker, Mark, and Emily Cochrane. 2020a. "Native American Tribes Sue Treasury over Stimulus Aid as They Feud over Funding." *New York Times*, May 1, 2020. https://www.nytimes.com/2020/05/01/us/politics/coronavirus-native-american-tribes-treasury-stimulus.html?searchResultPosition=25.

Walker, Mark, and Emily Cochrane. 2020b. "Tribe in South Dakota Seeks Court Ruling Over Standoff on Blocking Virus." *New York Times*, June 24, 2020. https://www.nytimes.com/2020/06/24/us/politics/coronavirus-south-dakota-tribe-standoff.html?searchResultPosition=7.

Warne, Donald, and Linda B. Frizzell. 2014. "American Indian Health Policy: Historical Trends and Contemporary Issues." *American Journal of Public Health* 104, no. S3: S263–57. https://doi.org/10.2105%2FAJPH.2013.301682.

Weimann, Gabriel, and Hans-Bernd Brosius. 2016. "A New Agenda for Agenda-Setting Research in the Digital Era." In *Political Communication in the Online World*, edited by G. Vowe and P. Henn, 26–44. New York: Routledge.

Weston, Mary Ann. 1996. *Native Americans in the News: Images of Indians in the Twentieth Century Press*. Westport, CT: Greenwood.

Wilkins, David E. 2016. "A History of Federal Indian Policy." In *Native American Voices*, 3rd ed., edited by Susan Lobo, Steve Talbot, and Traci L. Morris, 104–12. New York: Routledge.

Vizenor, Gerald Robert. 1999. *Manifest Manners: Narratives on Postindian Survivance*. Lincoln: University of Nebraska Press.

Yan, Wudan. 2020. "Remote and Ready to Fight Coronavirus's Next Wave." *New York Times*, May 16, 2020. https://www.nytimes.com/2020/05/16/health/coronavirus-vashon-washington.html?searchResultPosition=11.

LEGAL RESOURCES

Cherokee Nation v. Georgia, 30 U.S. 1 (1831)

Coronavirus Aid, Relief, and Economic Security (CARES) Act, Pub. L. No. 116–136, 134 Stat. 281 (2020)

Defense Production Act, Pub. L. No. 81–774, 64 Stat. 798 (1950)

Yellen v. Confederated Tribes of the Chehalis Reservation, S. Ct. 20–543 (2021)

PART III

COMMUNITY RESPONSES AND RESILIENCE

MARIANNE O. NIELSEN AND
KAREN JARRATT-SNIDER

I NDIGENOUS HEALTH ISSUES ARE interconnected, and resolutions, as mentioned in the introduction, are more holistic than those offered by Western medicine. Relationships are a key part of healing practices, and this includes relations not just between medical professionals and patients but with family members; community members; culture; and the living world around us, including nonhuman beings of all kinds (be they four-footed, eight-footed, not-footed, winged, or rooted), the earth and the sky, and the spirit world / spirituality.

In chapter 7, Thompson and Marek-Martinez describe how relations with the land are essential for the health and resilience of Indigenous Peoples, not just for practical reasons such as growing food, finding drinkable water, and harvesting medicinal plants but for a sense of identity and belonging, which are basic needs of all people. As Jarratt-Snider and Nielsen (2020) note, this deep connection to traditional homelands is one of the unique aspects of Indigenous environmental justice. In this volume, Thompson and Marek-Martinez discuss this connection in detail, which in turn explains why certain places and features of landscapes are considered culturally significant, or sacred, places. These authors demonstrate how connections to land are part of Indigenous health.

The Indian Removal Act of 1830 was the policy face of the American federal government's forced relocation policy that affected the majority of Indigenous Peoples in the eastern United States (though many Indigenous Peoples and individuals had already been forced off their land by settler colonists). These federal policies moved them to lands not their own and already occupied by other Indigenous Peoples. Those who managed to remain on their own lands still suffered the same hardships of marginalization resulting from colonial processes such as violence, disease, economic loss, and the kidnapping of their children.

Their resilience saved them, however, and continues to protect Indigenous Peoples from the continuing attempts of corporations, abetted by various levels of government, to remove them from their land and resources, and of governments to avoid providing the legally required (in the United States and Canada at least) financial support needed for adequate health-care services.

A great deal of health research about Indigenous Peoples focuses on the actions of communities and nations; very little focuses on the actual organizations that provide the services. This volume has two chapters that are the exception. First, Dietrich and Schroedel's chapter 2 in part I focuses on the issues that plague the Indian Health Service. Second, chapter 8 by Dodd and Nielsen discusses an organization that provides programs to prevent violent victimization, Tuu Oho Mai Services, and highlights a serious health issue in many Indigenous communities in many countries, as Robyn (2023), Luna-Gordinier (2023), Jones and de Heer (2023), and many others have pointed out. Duran and Duran (1995) trace such violence directly back to colonization, through the concept of intergenerational posttraumatic stress disorder, a predecessor of a similar concept, historical trauma (HT). Brave Heart et al. (2011, 283) define HT as "cumulative emotional and psychological wounding across generations, including the lifespan, which emanates from massive group trauma," such as that caused by colonization. An important consequence of defining colonization impacts in such terms is that it empowers survivors and decreases isolation and a perception of being stigmatized (Brave Heart et al. 2011, 283). Brave Heart et al. conclude that in order for healing to occur, it is necessary to "restore and empower Indigenous Peoples, to reclaim our traditional selves, our traditional knowledge, and our right to be who we are and should be as healthy, vital, and vibrant communities, unencumbered by depression, overwhelming grief, substance abuse, and traumatic responses. In essence, we strive to transcend our collective traumatic past" (283).

Chapter 8 focuses on how Tuu Oho Mai works to provide more effective services for its Indigenous clients through the incorporation of spirituality and culture. Their strategies have the potential to provide templates for Indigenous organizations working to increase the effectiveness of their health programs to enhance not only the health but the resilience of their clients. It should be noted that innovative strategies occur worldwide among Indigenous organizations, not just in Aotearoa / New Zealand. The program centers on the use of Māori culture and spirituality to help in healing those who suffer from family violence and those who perpetrate it. Indigenous values, history, roles, and practices are taught as a means to prevent further domestic violence and increase the resilience of the participants. As Lewis et al. (2021, 987) write about a long-running Cherokee program intended to heal historical trauma, "Teaching tribally-specific historical events was related to increased thoughts about historical loss, an increased awareness of non-Native people's lack of historical knowledge about Native people and subsequent experiences of discrimination, but also an increased sense of tribal identity, resilience, and belonging."

Spirituality and culture are not usually seen as parts of Western medicine, but they are central to Indigenous healing practices. To heal any relationships, including those originating in issues of justice—whether it is justice between individuals, between governments and Indigenous nations, or between corporations and Indigenous lands and resources—cultural resources are relied upon (see Jarratt-Snider and Nielsen 2020 and Nielsen and Jarratt-Snider 2018 for examples). Ross (2014, 10–11), discussing healing and the contrast between the concept of justice among Canadian Indigenous Peoples and non-Indigenous peoples, writes that if

> your way of knowing focuses on relationships rather than individual people, it will be natural to see that the relationships between human, animal, plant and earth/water aspects of Creation are fundamentally those of dependency. Once you do that, everything changes. We become, in our own eyes, dependent on the health of everything else. Our obligation then must be to promote accommodation with, rather than to seek dominance over, all things. A justice system must work to restore accommodation where relationships have been broken, not promote further alienation between people.

In just this way, justice is linked by the authors in this section to the health of Indigenous Peoples.

REFERENCES

Brave Heart, Maria Yellow Horse, Josephine Chase, Jennifer Elkins, and Deborah B. Altschul. 2011. "Historical Trauma Among Indigenous Peoples of the Americas: Concepts, Research, and Clinical Consideration." *Journal of Psychoactive Drugs* 43, no. 4: 282–90. https://doi.org/10.1080/02791072.2011.628913.

Duran, Eduardo, and Bonnie Duran. 1995. *Native American Postcolonial Psychology*. New York: SUNY Press.

Jarratt-Snider, Karen, and Marianne O. Nielsen, eds. 2020. *Indigenous Environmental Justice*. Tucson: University of Arizona Press.

Jones, Lynn C., and Brooke de Heer. 2023. "Gender, Health, and Justice Among Two-Spirit People." In *Indigenous Justice and Gender*, edited by Marianne O. Nielsen and Karen Jarratt-Snider, 61–77. Tucson: University of Arizona Press.

Lewis, Melissa, Rose Stremlau, Melissa Walls, Julie Reed, Jack Baker, Wyman Kirk, and Tom Belt. 2021. "Psychosocial Aspects of Historical and Cultural Learning: Historical Trauma and Resilience Among Indigenous Young Adults." *Journal of Health Care for the Poor and Underserved* 32: 987–1018. https://doi.org/10.1353/hpu.2021.0076.

Luna-Gordinier, Anne. 2023. "Restoring Tribal Jurisdiction with the Violence Against Women Act." In *Indigenous Justice and Gender*, edited by Marianne O. Nielsen and Karen Jarratt-Snider, 83–103. Tucson: University of Arizona Press.

Nielsen, Marianne O., and Karen Jarratt-Snider, eds. 2018. *Crime and Social Justice in Indian Country*. Tucson: University of Arizona Press.

Robyn, Linda M. 2023. "Missing and Murdered Indigenous Women and Girls: Strengthening Safety in Indian Country." In *Indigenous Justice and Gender*, edited by Marianne O. Nielsen and Karen Jarratt-Snider, 105–30. Tucson: University of Arizona Press.

Ross, Rupert. 2014. *Indigenous Healing: Exploring Traditional Paths*. Toronto: Penguin.

LEGAL RESOURCES

Indian Removal Act, Pub. L. No. 21–148, 4 Stat. 411 (1830)

7

REMAKING PLACE

Diné Land, Health, and Wellness

KERRY F. THOMPSON AND
ORA V. MAREK-MARTINEZ

THE HEALTH OF THE DINÉ[1] landscape called Diné Bikeyah is critical to Diné health. Cultural resources in the form of traditional cultural places (TCPs), plant-gathering areas, and archaeological sites are important components of the Diné landscape. While Diné interactions with archaeological sites center on avoidance, many Diné are engaged with TCPs and plant-gathering areas throughout Diné Bikeyah. The general health of the land and maintaining its viability for future generations is also a concern (Necefer et al. 2015). An organizing principle of the Diné universe, ké, confers an inescapable state of interrelatedness, interconnectedness, and interdependence among all things (Austin 2009, 83). Negative or disharmonious actions by one actor can, and do, reverberate throughout the entire system of ké. The boundaries of the more than twenty-seven-thousand-square-mile Navajo Nation do not enclose or hem in the system of ké and they do not define the extent to which Diné relationships with the land continue to exist. The reservation is part of the homeland to which Diné maintain access, however, and intimate connections to all Diné Bikeyah are maintained through oral tradition, ceremonial practices, and pilgrimage. Today, though, like many others, the Navajo Nation is grappling with significant health issues among its

---

1. *Diné* and *Navajo* are often used interchangeably. We will use *Diné* unless referencing work, or entities that specifically use *Navajo* like *Navajo Wellness Model* or *Navajo Nation*.

population in addition to social challenges that inhibit the teaching and learning of healthy relationships among Diné and their land.

Oral traditions connect people to landscapes because people attach significance to places, and places in turn become core pieces of a group's identity (Basso 1996). Natural features often have cultural meanings for inhabitants of a landscape (Crumley 1999; Knapp and Ashmore 1999; Lovis and Whallon 2016). Indigenous cultures around the world often map their worlds through lived experience (Bender 1999). An Indigenous group's world map will include places of significance with histories that are anchored spatially, remembered mnemonically, and transmitted orally (Bender 1999; Crumley 1999). The geography remembered in oral traditions is also important for maintaining cultural institutions.

There are many examples of published oral traditions that relate the significance of Diné Bikeyah (e.g., Haile 1979; Kluckhohn 1944, 158–74; Wyman 1970). Aside from the actual telling of the oral traditions themselves, the emphasis on geographic knowledge via the oral tradition (and the administration of geography tests to individuals within the traditions) highlights the meaningfulness of the landscape in Diné culture. The Blessingway, for example, contains a song in which a guessing technique is introduced, whereby a question of location is posed and in the next song, the answer is given—these songs emphasize that importance of knowing the sacred mountains and their locations (Wyman 1970, 158). In another tradition, the Sun administers a test of his twin sons' knowledge of the four mountains and the San Juan River and Rio Grande to gauge the sons' worthiness to wield a particular weapon (O'Bryan 1956, 82). Researchers have also variously commented on the attention to geography and movement among Diné and in their oral traditions. Wyman (1962, 78), for example, writes, "Much has been said about the Navaho's [*sic*] passion for geography, his preoccupation with locality, and what is probably more important, his high evaluation of moving from place to place," and Newcomb and Reichard ([1937] 1975, 69) observe that "locality is of the greatest importance to the Navajo people." As with many Indigenous Peoples, health among Diné cannot be separated from the land and its resources. Understanding the landscape through the continued transmission of oral tradition is the primary means through which younger Diné may forge and maintain a mutually beneficial relationship with the land and safeguard their own health.

In recent years, we have seen a diverse range of Indigenous health, well-being, and wellness initiatives increase on both mainstream social media platforms, such as Instagram, YouTube, and TikTok, and within Indigenous communities. Such initiatives span from physical wellness to emotional wellness, and they tend to lean toward efforts to heal from trauma, experienced either intergenerationally or contemporarily, through the use of ancestral cultural practices. Through land-based initiatives, Indigenous communities have sought to restore, reclaim, and maintain health and well-being as well as reconnect to their communities and homelands. These initiatives have focused on how to nurture individual and communal relationships with the land. The landscape is embedded with cultural meaning and sacred sites, ceremonial sites, and other culturally significant sites that are "an integral and inseparable part of the entire culture" (Marek-Martinez 2016, 53). These land-based connections then assist in reconnecting with one's family and community, as this information is usually shared through oral traditions. Coming to know the land is a way to know your People, your history, your connections, and yourself; reestablishing a connection with the land has always been a way to maintain health and well-being.

In this chapter, we discuss the remaking of Diné places on the cultural landscape to assist with maintaining and achieving good health and wellness, which includes relearning and reconnecting with the land and our relatives. We are two Diné *asdzáán* (Navajo women) who have been involved in the protection of Diné cultural heritage and lands in various ways through our work in archaeology. As a child growing up on the Nez Perce Reservation in Idaho, I (Marek-Martinez) was introduced to the protocols associated with the cultural landscape that held our language, our histories, and our ancestors. These protocols provided me with the skills to live in our cultural homelands and to respect and honor the relationships we cultivate with the land and within our community. Learning about the role of women in the community meant learning about locating, gathering, and caring for our cultural foods in order to ensure they would provide for future generation; in other words, we enacted "perpetuation" of our cultural foods through these everyday processes (Corntassel and Hardbarger 2019, 89). These lessons also taught me the value and importance of reciprocity and interdependence as means of maintaining healthy relationships with the landscape and within the community. My (Thompson) connection to our land is through the sheepherding, farming, and playing I did as a kid. After many, many years away, I returned to live in my home community on the Navajo reservation ten years ago. In the last ten years, I have walked the landscape where I grew up, built a home, and tried to return to the farming I knew as a child. I learn about plants and soil from books and knowledgeable friends, and on my walks, I observe the fluctuating health of the river valley in which we live. The knowledge I have is incomplete, but remaking my place is a lengthy process.

DINÉ PHILOSOPHY AND WELLNESS MODELS

There are two models that stand out in the literature on Navajo health. The first, called the Navajo Wellness Model, was developed by the Navajo Area Indian Health Service in partnership with Diné cultural experts, philosophers, and traditional healers as part of a curriculum called Shá'bek'ehgo As'ah Oodááł: A Journey with Wellness and Healthy Lifestyle Guided by the Journey of the Sun (Nelson 2018). The second, called the Diné Hózhó Resilience Model, derives from the Hózhó Wellness Philosophy and was developed through the analysis of the concept of *hózhó*, first, and then secondary analysis of preexisting data from the Centers for American Indian and Alaska Native Health (Kahn-John and Koithan 2015). Both models are also depicted visually using culturally referent symbols.

The Navajo Wellness Model (NWM) emphasizes four domains of health: self-identity, self-respect, self-care, and protection of self as necessary for a core of resilience. Personal and family health, healthy communities, and a healthy environment are to be achieved through the attention to daily exercise, healthy eating, and maintaining a balance in all aspects of life organized *sa bik'ehgo*, or sunwise—to follow the natural order of the day and of life (Nelson 2018). The image in Nelson of NWM is of the four domains of health arranged around resilience within the four sacred mountains that define the Diné landscape, or *hooghan*—home place. At the top of the illustration in the opening of the larger *hooghan*, is the domain of self-identity (Nelson 2018).

Articulating the Hózhó Wellness Philosophy, Kahn-John (2010) explains that healthy relationships, or *ké*, are a key component of personal, family, community, and environmental health. Relationships, however, represent but one of six concepts (Kahn-John 2010) that characterize the Diné philosophy of *hózhó*. As Austin (2009, 54) explains, "Hózhó encompasses everything that Navajos consider positive and good; positive characteristics that Navajos believe contribute to living life to the fullest. These positive characteristics include beauty, harmony, goodness, happiness, right social relations, good health, and acquisition of knowledge." The other concepts that characterize *hózhó* include spirituality, respect, reciprocity, discipline, and thinking (Kahn-John 2010), and all are key components to the Hózhó Wellness Philosophy (Kahn-John and Koithan 2015). The philosophy also emphasizes responsible thought, speech, and behavior as pathways to self-empowerment (Kahn-John and Koithan 2015). The Diné Hózhó Resilience Model (HRM), developed from the philosophy, comprises three domains: harmony, respect, and spirituality. The domains are depicted as projectile points (arrowheads), with lines that illustrate their interconnectedness with each other and with the centrally placed concept of resilience, on a circular backdrop with a rainbow opened to the top of the figure, where the domain of harmony is placed (Kahn-John and Koithan 2015).

Each model is made up of interconnected domains—four in NWM and three in HRM—all of which are arranged around the concept of resilience. Both models specifically center the natural world as crucial to Diné health and well-being and use cultural references to landscapes to illustrate domains of health. NWM uses the four sacred mountains and the idea of *hooghan*, illustrated as an octagonal structure in the style of what is called a hogan in English. The HRM depiction of landscape is more abstract. The circular but not enclosed rainbow opening to the top of the image seems to reference the band on a Diné wedding basket that symbolizes the earth. The placement of harmony at the opening of the rainbow in HRM and the similar placement of self-identity at the doorway of the *hooghan* in NWM signify together both the individual and communal orientations of Diné culture. According to Austin (2009, 55), "Navajos value an individualism that is tempered by reciprocal duties and obligations to relatives, kinfolks, and people in general." The respect for self is an integral part of both models because without it, harmony cannot be built.

INDIGENOUS-BASED WELLNESS INITIATIVES

The increase in Indigenous-based wellness initiatives has also resulted in models that resonate with many different Indigenous Peoples' philosophies, taking more of a generalized approach to health and wellness. The Well for Culture Indigenous Wellness Initiative, formed by cofounders Thosh Collins (Onk-Akimel O'odham, Wa-Zha-Zhi, Haudenosaunee) and Chelsey Luger (Lakota, Ojibwe), focuses on a holistic model called the Seven Circles of Wellness that "encourages wellness among Indigenous people in order to sustain, rebuild, and strengthen our communities" (Well for Culture, n.d.). Their impetus for creating the model was to encourage health and well-being among Indigenous people using ancestral knowledge to begin reconnecting to Indigenous wellness. They emphasize seven interconnected circles of ancestral components of health and well-being—sleep, real food, movement, kinship/clanship/community, connection to earth, sacred space, and stress management—which they identified through intensive interviews and time spent in various Indigenous communities.

Collins and Luger (Well for Culture, n.d.) center community knowledge, which is a storied compendium of the varied individual and collective experiences that Indigenous community members hold, as key determinants of reclaiming and rebuilding strong and healthy communities. In their model, they advocate for becoming trauma-informed as a way to understand the larger and complex landscape of Indigenous issues and how they impact Indigenous Peoples in both indirect and direct ways, as well as intergenerationally. Learning about and understanding the trauma experienced by a community or a family, and how an individual is a part of this trauma, is essential to the healing process and to overall health and well-being. An important aspect of their model is understanding that for the vast majority of Indigenous Peoples' history, they were healthy, strong, and active, and it wasn't until the entrance of settler colonizers that this began to change. Colonization of Indigenous Peoples at the hands of settler governments began with disconnecting them from their ancestral homelands, which forced a separation from the people to their way of life and to the spiritual connections that Indigenous Peoples maintain with their landscapes (Well for Culture, n.d.).

This focus on landscapes and ancestral knowledge leading to wellness is an inherent aspect of many Indigenous cultures. As part of Well for Culture's overall vision, they acknowledge the power and value of ancestral knowledge to achieving and maintaining wellness today. They understand wellness through an Indigenous lens of interconnectedness that begins to create a sense of relationality and balance in all aspects of life, which is achieved and nurtured through relationships with the land. The continuation of adaptive practices by Indigenous Peoples, the assimilation of new knowledge and information into culture and practice, is a strategy enacted to overcome the detrimental effects of colonization and its impact on Indigenous Peoples' wellness; braiding ancestral knowledge and new knowledge creates "an ongoing chain of knowledge" (Well for Culture, n.d.) that perpetuates ancestral knowledge and relationships with the land.

LAND AS A DETERMINANT OF HEALTH

Humans give meaning to and form relationships with their surroundings. Humans inscribe their presence on their surroundings and form meaningful relationships with the locales that they occupy (Low and Lawrence-Zúñiga 2003; Rodman 2003). People attach significance to places and places, in turn, become core pieces of a group's identity (Basso 1996). Colonization disrupted relationships among Indigenous Peoples, their kin, and their land (Greenwood and Lindsay 2019; Hansen 2018). The impact of settler colonialism on the relationships of Indigenous Peoples with their lands has been wholly negative, resulting in significant health disparities, among other issues (Ahmed, Zuk, and Tsuji 2021).

Geography is, itself, a determinant of Indigenous health that stands apart from other social determinants of health (de Leeuw 2018). Because space and place are active forces in human existence (de Leeuw 2018), understanding the impact of environmental dispossession on Indigenous Peoples is a crucial factor in understanding Indigenous health outcomes (Ahmed, Zuk, and Tsuji 2021; Richmond 2018). Exploitation by land-based, extractive industries is not only unhealthy for the physical body, but it also has negative outcomes on the practice and efficacy of ceremonies (Begay 2001; Corntassel and Hardbarger 2019). The Western framework of health emphasizes the absence of disease in the body (Parlee, Berkes, and the Teetl'it Gwich'in 2005). Landscape and people in Indigenous conceptions of health and well-being, however, are inseparable (Begay 2001; de Leeuw 2018; Greenwood and Lindsay 2019; Parlee, Berkes, and the Teetl'it Gwich'in 2005; Nelson 2020; Richmond 2018; Schultz et al. 2018).

Indigenous languages and cultural practices are embedded in the landscape, composed of multiple dimensions, such as the spiritual, emotional, and intellectual aspects, which support renewing and reclaiming relationships with the land and community (Fast et al. 2021; Corntassel and Hardbarger 2019). The holistic nature of land-based pedagogy enables learners to not only learn practical skills like hunting, fishing, and gathering, but it also teaches cultural values, ethics, and reciprocity (Simpson 2014). Indigenous protocols with respect to the land are created intentionally with the purpose to teach these values and ethics and to demonstrate the delicate balance that exists in nature. In learning these protocols, Indigenous Peoples are interconnected with their ancestors, with their relatives, and with their culture.

CONCLUSION

Land-based pedagogy as a decolonizing project aims to reconnect Indigenous Peoples with their land and thus improve other areas of Indigenous life (Wildcat et al. 2014); it is also about the act of reclaiming relationships that are grounded in the land and in the community (Corntassel and Hardbarger 2019). Deloria and Wildcat explain that an "Indigenous metaphysics" is the understanding that humans are one small part of "an immense complex living system," wherein humans are interconnected, related, and dependent on other beings and the elements (2001, 12; see also Ahmed, Zuk, and Tsuji 2021). Our existence as humans is also bound to the wellness and health of other beings and places, and within these places exists a power invoked by experiences in a particular place. Land-based pedagogy is described as a way of learning and teaching from the land "that has existed since the beginning of humans"; it is also becoming an active demonstration of respect and acknowledgement of Indigenous and Western knowledge systems (Canadian Commission for UNESCO 2021; see also Deloria and Wildcat 2001), a sort of dialectical relationship between these two disparate knowledge systems.

Indigenous Peoples continue to renew, relearn, and reestablish relationships with the land and their communities, through acts of "ceremony, resurgence, presence, and rearticulation" (Tuck and Habtom 2019, 243). The interconnection and interrelatedness that Indigenous Peoples enact with the cultural landscape has resulted in a reclamation and resurgence of ancestral knowledges akin to decolonization methodologies that are meant to restore, revitalize, and reconnect Indigenous Peoples with their homelands, families, and communities, both animate and inanimate (Ahmed, Zuk, and Tsuji 2021; Corntassel and Hardbarger 2019; Hansen 2018; Maunakea 2021; Simpson 2014; Wildcat et al. 2014). Through the lens of Indigenous health and wellness frameworks, we begin to see that the land, and how it is treated, is an embodiment of the treatment of Indigenous Peoples within settler-colonizer states. Thus the disconnection of Indigenous Peoples from their lands at the hand of colonization has contributed to the decline in health and wellness that we currently see within Indigenous communities.

REFERENCES

Ahmed, Fatima, Aleksandra M. Zuk, and Leonard J. S. Tsuji. 2021. "The Impact of Land-Based Physical Activity Interventions on Self-Reported Health and Well-Being of Indigenous Adults: A Systematic Review." *International Journal of Environmental Research and Public Health* 18, no. 13: 1–23. https://doi.org/10.3390/ijerph18137099.

Austin, Raymond D. 2009. *Navajo Courts and Navajo Common Law: A Tradition of Tribal Self-Governance*. Minneapolis: University of Minnesota Press.

Basso, Keith H. 1996. *Wisdom Sits in Places: Landscape and Language Among the Western Apache*. Albuquerque: University of New Mexico Press.

Begay, Robert M. 2001. "Doo Dilzin Da: 'Abuse of the Natural World.'" *American Indian Quarterly* 25, no. 1: 21–27. https://www.jstor.org/stable/1186002.

Bender, Barbara. 1999. "Subverting the Western Gaze: Mapping Alternative Worlds." In *The Archaeology and Anthropology of Landscape: Shaping Your Landscape*, edited by Peter J. Ucko and Robert Layton, 31–45. London: Routledge.

Canadian Commission for UNESCO. 2021. "Land as Teacher: Understanding Indigenous Land-Based Education." June 21, 2021. https://en.ccunesco.ca /idealab/indigenous-land-based-education.

Corntassel, Jeff, and Tiffanie Hardbarger. 2019. "Educate to Perpetuate: Land-Based Pedagogies and Community Resurgence." *International Review of Education* 65: 87–116. https://doi.org/10.1007/s11159-018-9759-1.

Crumley, Carole L. 1999. "Sacred Landscapes: Constructed and Conceptualized." In *Archaeologies of Landscape: Contemporary Perspectives*, edited by Wendy Ashmore and A. Bernard Knapp, 269–76. Malden, MA: Blackwell Publishing.

de Leeuw, Sarah. 2018. "Activating Place: Geography as a Determinant of Indigenous Peoples' Health and Well-Being." In *Determinants of Indigenous Peoples' Health: Beyond the Social*, 2nd ed., edited by Margo Greenwood, Sarah de Leeuw, and Nicole Marie Lindsay, 187–203. Toronto: Canadian Scholars.

Deloria, Vine, Jr., and Daniel R. Wildcat. 2001. *Power and Place: Indian Education in America*. Golden, CO: American Indian Graduate Center and Fulcrum Resources.

Fast, Elizabeth, Melanie Lefebrve, Christopher Reid, Brooke Wahsontiiostha Deer, Dakota Swiftwolfe, Moe Clark, Vicky Boldo, Juliet Mackie, Rupert Mackie, and Karen Tutanuak. 2021. "Restoring Our Roots: Land-Based Community by and for Indigenous Youth." *International Journal of Indigenous Health* 16, no. 2: 120–38. https://doi.org/10.32799/ijih.v16i2.33932.

Greenwood, Margo, and Nicole Marie Lindsay. 2019. "A Commentary on Land, Health, and Indigenous Knowledge(s)." *Global Health Promotion* 26, no. S3: S82–86. https://doi.org/10.1177/1757975919831262.

Haile, Berard. 1979. *Waterway*. Flagstaff: Museum of Northern Arizona Press.

Hansen, John. 2018. "Cree Elders' Perspectives on Land-Based Education: A Case Study." *Brock Education Journal* 28, no. 1: 74–91. https://doi.org/10.26522 /brocked.v28i1.783.

Kahn-John, Michelle. 2010. "Concept Analysis of Diné Hózhó: A Diné Wellness Philosophy." *Advances in Nursing Science* 33, no. 2: 113–25. https://doi.org/10 .1097/ans.0b013e3181dbc658.

Kahn-John, Michelle, and Mary Koithan. 2015. "Living in Health, Harmony, and Beauty: The Diné (Navajo) Hózhó Wellness Philosophy." *Global Advances in Health and Medicine* 4, no. 3 (May): 24–30. https://doi.org/10.7453%2Fgahmj .2015.044.

Kluckhohn, Clyde. 1944. *Navaho Witchcraft*. Papers of the Peabody Museum of American Archaeology and Ethnology, Harvard University, vol. XXII, no. 2. Cambridge, MA: Harvard University.

Knapp, A. Bernard, and Wendy Ashmore, eds. 1999. "Archaeological Landscapes: Constructed, Conceptualized, Ideational." In *Archaeologies of Landscape: Contemporary Perspectives*, edited by Wendy Ashmore and A. Bernard Knapp, 1–30. Malden: Blackwell Publishing.

Lovis, William A., and Robert Whallon. 2016. "The Creation of Landscape Meaning by Mobile Hunter-Gatherers." In *Marking the Land: Hunter-Gatherer Creation of Meaning in Their Environment*, edited by William A. Lovis and Robert Whallon, 1–9. New York: Routledge.

Low, Setha M., and Denise Lawrence-Zúñiga. 2003. *The Anthropology of Space and Place: Locating Culture*. Malden, MA: Blackwell Publishing.

Marek-Martinez, Ora V. 2016. "Archaeology for, by, and with the Navajo People: The Nihookáá Dine'é' Bila'Ashdla'ii Way." PhD diss., University of California, Berkeley. https://escholarship.org/uc/item/6w9792rg.

Maunakea, Summer P. 2021. "Toward a Framework for Āina-Based Pedagogies: A Hawai'i Approach to Indigenous Land-Based Education." *Journal of Higher Education Theory & Practice* 21, no. 10: 278–86. https://doi.org/10.33423/jhetp.v21i10.4641.

Necefer, Len, Gabrielle Wong-Parodi, Paulina Jaramillo, Mitchell J. Small. 2015. "Energy Development and Native Americans: Values and Beliefs about Energy from the Navajo Nation." *Energy Research & Social Science* 7 (May): 1–11. https://doi.org/10.1016/j.erss.2015.02.007.

Nelson, Marie. 2018. *Navajo Wellness Model: Keeping the Cultural Teachings Alive to Improve Health*. Indian Health Service Blog. January 4, 2018. https://www.ihs.gov/newsroom/ihs-blog/january2018/navajo-wellness-model-keeping-the-cultural-teachings-alive-to-improve-health/.

Nelson, Peter A. 2020. "Refusing Settler Epistemologies and Maintaining an Indigenous Future of Tolay Lake, Sonoma County, California." *American Indian Quarterly* 44, no. 2: 221–42. https://doi.org/10.5250/amerindiquar.44.2.0221.

Newcomb, Franc Johnson, and Gladys Reichard. (1937) 1975. *Sandpaintings of the Navajo Shooting Chant*. New York: J. J. Augustin. Reprint, New York: Dover. Citations refer to the Dover edition.

O'Bryan, Aileen. 1956. "The Diné: Origin Myths of the Navaho Indians." *Bureau of American Ethnology Bulletin* 163: 1–194. Washington, D.C.: Smithsonian Institution. https://repository.si.edu/handle/10088/15457.

Parlee, Brenda, Fikret Berkes, and the Teetl'it Gwich'in. 2005. "Health of the Land, Health of the People: A Case Study on Gwich'in Berry Harvesting in Northern Canada." *EcoHealth* 2: 127–37. https://link.springer.com/article/10.1007/s10393-005-3870-z.

Richmond, Chantelle. 2018. "The Relatedness of People, Land, and Health: Stories from Anishinabe Elders." In *Determinants of Indigenous Peoples' Health: Beyond the Social*, 2nd ed., edited by Margo Greenwood, Sarah de Leeuw, Nicole Marie Lindsay, 167–86. Toronto: Canadian Scholars.

Rodman, Margaret C. 2003. "Empowering Place: Multilocality and Multivocality." In *The Anthropology of Space and Place: Locating Culture*, edited by Setha M. Low and Denise Lawrence-Zúñiga, 204–23. Malden, MA: Blackwell Publishing.

Schultz, Rosalie, Tammy Abott, Jessica Yamaguchi, and Sheree Cairney. 2018. "Indigenous Land Management as Primary Health Care: Qualitative Analysis from the Interplay Research in Remote Australia." *BMC Health Services Research* 18: 960–70. https://doi.org/10.1186/s12913-018-3764-8.

Simpson, Leanne Betasamosake. 2014. "Land as Pedagogy: Nishnaabeg Intelligence and Rebellious Transformation." *Decolonization: Indigeneity, Education & Society* 3, no. 3: 1–25. https://jps.library.utoronto.ca/index.php/des/article/view/22170/17985.

Tuck, Eve, and Sefanit Habtom. 2019. "Unforgetting Place in Urban Education Through Creative Participatory Visual Methods." *Educational Theory* 69, no. 2: 241–56. https://doi.org/10.1111/edth.12366.

Well for Culture. n.d. "Home." Accessed December 22, 2021. https://www.wellforculture.com/.

Wildcat, Matthew, Mandee McDonald, Stephanie Irlbacher-Fox, and Glen Coulthard. 2014. "Learning from the Land: Indigenous Land Based Pedagogy and Decolonization." *Decolonization: Indigeneity, Education & Society* 3, no. 3: i–xv. https://jps.library.utoronto.ca/index.php/des/article/view/22248/18062.

Wyman, Leland. 1962. *The Windways of the Navaho*. Colorado Springs: Taylor Museum of the Colorado Fine Arts Center.

Wyman, Leland. 1970. *Blessingway*. Tucson: University of Arizona Press.

8

RESTORING MANA

How One Māori Agency Is Addressing Domestic Violence

KANOELANI R. DODD AND MARIANNE O. NIELSEN

W HEN DOING RESEARCH ON the health and resilience of Indigenous Peoples, it is necessary to focus not just on Indigenous individuals and communities but on the Indigenous
organizations that enable Indigenous Peoples to practice de facto sovereignty by providing much-needed culturally sensitive, appropriate, and
accessible health services that may be otherwise lacking. Just as Indigenous communities face challenges in overcoming the impacts of settler
colonialism, so do these organizations. Their survival can literally be a
matter of life and death to their Indigenous clients in need.

In this chapter, we provide a case study of Tuu Oho Mai Services,
formerly known as the Hamilton Abuse Intervention Project (HAIP),
which for thirty years has been serving those harmed and doing harm
in domestic violence cases in Aotearoa (New Zealand). The description
of the agency is based, first, on face-to-face interviews done in 2002 by
Nielsen, which were extensively updated via Zoom and secondary sources
by Dodd in 2022. This update was with the permission and collaboration
of Mr. Poata Watene, the CEO of Tuu Oho Mai, who not only provided
extensive information about the growth and philosophy of the agency but
reviewed the chapter for accuracy before publication. We are extremely
grateful for his assistance and enthusiasm in sharing the factors contributing to the organization's resilience and good work.

At the time of its launch in 1991, HAIP was designed after a mainstream American treatment model, with the aim of addressing domestic violence in Māori and non-Māori households by strengthening the *whānau* (family). Although the purpose remains the same, Tuu Oho Mai has transitioned its approaches to better serve its Māori and other Oceanian populations, which make up more than half of its clientele. In doing so, it serves as an example of the resilience of Māori service-providers and organizations in adapting to a changing settler colonial environment.

This chapter discusses characteristics of the organization, including historical changes in its services and philosophy. Our primary goal is to demonstrate the importance of Indigenous organizations having the autonomy to create their own programs and operations in order to address systemic community health issues arising from settler colonialism. To understand the importance of Tuu Oho Mai's services, it is necessary to understand some of the history of Aotearoa / New Zealand. For that reason, we briefly describe settler colonialism in Aotearoa as context for the current conditions in which Māori continue to live. As well, we frequently use *te reo Māori* (Māori language) throughout this chapter. It is important to breathe life into speech, as is done when Indigenous people use their Indigenous languages. Whether words or place-names, such usage actively decolonizes spaces. *Te reo Māori*, like so many other Indigenous languages, was predicted to go extinct as a consequence of colonization, yet, through revitalization efforts, the language thrives once more. We will also use the inclusive term *Oceanian*, which includes Polynesians, Micronesians, and Melanesians, where appropriate.

SETTLER COLONIALISM IN AOTEAROA

Aotearoa is the Indigenous name for New Zealand. The colonial name came about when Dutch explorer Abel Tasman in 1642 decided to honor the Dutch province of Zeeland. The very mapping of Oceania, to which he contributed, served as a "tool of colonial domination" (Mezzadra and Neilson 2013, 15). Ultimately, the creation of these subregions put in place a racial hierarchy that divided groups of people who share similar ancestry, languages, and culture.

MĀORI SETTLEMENT

The peopling of Oceania is well documented in chants and oral histories (Coates 2004). Māori origins speak of a distant land of Hawaiki, which isn't a specific location in Oceania but rather a term that means "homeland" (Walker 1990). Exactly when Māori settled Aotearoa is not clear. Walker (1990) notes settlement occurred around AD 800. King (1992) speculates that settlement occurred in waves, beginning between AD 500 and 800 until AD 1350. The definitive reasons for migrating from Hawaiki to Aotearoa are unknown, but migration was certainly purposeful. Māori, like their other Oceanian relatives, are at home with the sea, as explained by Hau'ofa (1994).

Historically, Māori society consisted of *whānau* (family), *hapū* (subtribe), and *iwi* (tribe). The *whānau* consisted of immediate and extended family and was the core of society. As *whānau* grew over time, the group "would be elevated to the status of hapū" (Walker 1990, 64). As *whānau* grew into *hapū* and finally *iwi*, life within Māori society grew more complex. This complexity was mediated by *mana*, a central element of Māori life.

Mana was a staple element of Māori identity. Although *mana* can be translated to "spiritual authority," "status," and "sovereignty," the term is complex, as individuals, communities, and places all have *mana*. As captured in the words of Durie (1998, 2), "Mana has both worldly and ethereal meaning." *Mana* predates colonization; it is an ancient concept that cannot be fully appreciated using the English language or Western ideology. For the purpose of this chapter, Dodd's interpretation of *mana*, based on the work of Walker (1990), Durie (1998), and Trask (1999), can be understood as one's physical and spiritual authority, which connects them to the land, ancestors, community, cosmos, and self.

Mana was obscured as colonial ideologies were deemed superior by the settler colonists. As stated by Balzer (1999, 243), "The existence of Indigenous culture and the right to self-determination were subsumed under British imperialism." *Mana* ensured Māori relations within the universe, and with the destruction of those relations, violence increased. It is then in restoring one's *mana* that the balancing of self (*hanau*) and community begins to take place.

COLONIAL CONTEXT

After nearly eight hundred years of Māori settlement, the first Pākehā (Europeans) landed in Aotearoa (Walker 1990) with the arrival of explorer Abel Tasman. Tasman's first contact with the Māori turned fatal when his men responded to the sounding of the *pūtātara* (conch shell) with their horns. In an attempt to mirror the Māori, the Dutch unknowingly challenged them instead (Fischer 2002). This altercation resulted in the death of a few of Tasman's men. Tasman consequently labeled the Māori as savage and barbaric (Salmond 1997). After the Tasman affair, it would be over one hundred years until the next foreigner would arrive.

Captain James Cook made landfall in Aotearoa in 1769. In the less than one hundred years after Cook's arrival, Māori endured waves of change as Pākehā sought occupied land and valuable natural resources. Smith (2005) notes that some of the earliest tools of colonizing Aotearoa were the development of hierarchies informed by colonial ideologies rooted in patriarchy. Colonial ideologies altered definitions of gender and family. Those alterations debilitated individual and communal *mana*. As stated by Ross (2014, 77), "The removal of women from positions of power and authority was an important step in colonization."

Traditionally, Māori women held diverse roles as warriors, leaders, master artists, educators, and creators of life. The devaluing of Māori women and their societal roles was used to justify rape, exploitation, and violence (Nielsen and Robyn 2019). Moreover, violence was utilized as a tool to maintain capitalist social systems (Erai 2020). Although domestic violence was not exclusive to colonial contact, traditional mechanisms of control to address such offenses deteriorated with colonization. Domestic violence, in particular, "was legal in all British colonies during early-mid colonial periods" (Nielsen and Robyn 2019, 117).

In addition to the subordination of Māori women, Māori men were stripped of their traditional roles as warriors, protectors, leaders, and fathers (Duran and Duran 1995). Land and role dispossession interrelated as Pākehā custom and ideology superseded traditional Māori life.

Ultimately, the dispossession of land and societal roles correlates with the internalization and externalization of violence (Nielsen and Robyn 2019). Unfortunately, the alienation of Māori from their traditional lands and means of survival was sanctioned in the English version of the Treaty of Waitangi in 1840 (see Walker 1990).

DOMESTIC VIOLENCE IN AOTEAROA TODAY

Impacts stemming from colonization, both deliberate and unintentional, remain observable in numerous facets of Aotearoa today. High rates of domestic violence among Māori are one of them. In a three-cycle, face-to-face, random sample survey conducted between 2018 and 2020 with over seven thousand participants in each cycle, Māori were found to have experienced the highest rates of victimization of all ethnic groups (NZ Justice 2021). Māori women, in particular, are more than twice as likely to be victims of intimate partner violence than their Pākehā counterparts (Nielsen and Robyn 2019, 128). This statistic, alarming enough, has increased with the COVID-19 pandemic; research has shown that violence escalates and intensifies during times of emergencies as people experience strain (New Zealand Family Violence Clearinghouse 2022). The escalation of intimate partner violence amid the pandemic has impacted women around the globe and its prevalence has been coined the "Shadow Pandemic" (UN Women 2020). Statistics that capture the increase of intimate partner violence during the pandemic are still being produced, and research will likely continue well into the future.

Violence against Māori women has been an ongoing systemic issue, with collateral victims extending into the community. As Robertson (1999a; 1999b) points out, European and most colonized countries remain patriarchal. This fact is reflected in the laws, policies, and ideologies of the country's dominant class. When governments are slow in recognizing domestic violence as a severe offense, as seen in Aotearoa, the abuse tends to become normalized in communities. As the recognition of domestic violence and its severity increased in the communities of Aotearoa, pilot programs such as HAIP were developed.

DEVELOPMENT OF THE HAMILTON ABUSE INTERVENTION PROJECT (HAIP)

Settler colonialism set the stage for domestic violence issues and for the design and operation of service organizations established to deal with them. Such agencies were an Indigenous response to the institutional racism and patriarchy that dominated at the time (see Nielsen and Brown 2012). "New Zealand's government that institutionalized the denigration of things Māori and the devaluing of women is the same entity that Māori and Pākehā women must now turn to for protection from their batterers" (Balzer 1999, 247). The mistrust in the criminal justice and public health systems resulted in underreporting. Service organizations such as HAIP were developed to be innovative in their work to address and prevent future domestic violence.

HAIP was designed after the Duluth Model, which utilizes a dual response from the criminal justice system and the community (Balzer 1999, 239). The Duluth Model was groundbreaking when it was developed in 1981, as it was "the first practical programmatic approach to domestic violence that did not obscure or mask the historical realities" of colonization (Balzer 1999, 247). Further, the model challenged "historical victim-blaming narratives" (240).

At the time HAIP was established in the city of Hamilton, a mixed population of Māori and Pākehā was prevalent on the North Island. As noted by Balzer (1999, 241), a domestic violence steering committee was formed prior to the launch of HAIP in order to investigate the appropriateness of utilizing the Duluth Model. Upon approving the Duluth Model, one Pākehā and one Māori research team were then commissioned to examine the program's appropriateness for both ethnic groups. The Pākehā research team was the first to examine the project (Balzer 1999, 243–45), and they approved. The Māori team, on the other hand, "identified four factors of colonization that had a direct and causal impact on family violence: the denigration of *mana Māori*, the contradiction of the Treaty of Waitangi, breakdown of tribal structures and *whānau*, and the infiltration of an ideology of male supremacy on Māori consciousness" (245). Precisely what HAIP did to counteract these identified factors was unclear and may in part explain the eventual need for the program to transition to a model better fitted to serve its Māori population.

PURPOSE

The primary purpose of HAIP at the time of its development was unabashedly political: it was "to attempt to reform the New Zealand justice system's response to domestic violence, particularly the violence of men directed against their women partners" (Busch and Robertson 1994, 34). In the early stages of the pilot program, Balzer (1999, 251) asserts, "the notion that we should shift our focus from changing how individuals relate to being abused to how as a community we intervene was neither appreciated nor accepted by many." HAIP truly was groundbreaking in both its development and its ability to remain resilient in the face of public and governmental resistance.

Further, the aims of the organization in its beginning stage were "to co-ordinate family violence interventions in the Hamilton criminal justice area[;] to provide leadership endeavors to stop violence against women and their children, work towards the reduction of violence against women and their children, provide services and advocacy for battered women and their children, hold offenders accountable for their actions, be transparent in all activities[;] [and] to provide culturally appropriate responses in all areas HAIP works in" (HAIP 2001, 3). HAIP, which acted as a coordinating body, "brought together the women's refuges, the police, the criminal courts, the Family Court and the Probation Service" (Robertson 1999a, 217).

HISTORY OF HAIP

HAIP began its services in 1991 as a three-year national pilot project funded by the Family Violence Prevention Coordinating Committee. One reason the city of Hamilton was selected for the project was because of its high Māori population (Balzer 1999). HAIP was the first of its kind in Aotearoa and for many years provided the cutting edge of programming (anonymous participant 5, interview with Marianne O. Nielsen, November 29, 2002). HAIP was designed to prevent the high number of Māori in prison and to remind the male abusers of their obligations to their families and to future generations (anonymous participant 10, interview with Marianne O. Nielsen, November 27, 2002). Within the first two years of operation, HAIP served eight hundred men (Balzer 1999) and had contact with an unrecorded number of women.

In 1995, a government-commissioned review of HAIP "resulted in a downsizing of government involvement in the project and the end of the pilot period" (HAIP 2001, 3); the demonstration phase ended in 1996 (HAIP 2001). The federal government funding comprised about two-thirds of the agency's budget, so the organization had to restructure and maintain itself through various local community sources, including fee-for-service contracts with the municipal government and grants from the New Zealand Lottery Grants Board, private charitable foundations, and businesses. These funders included the Family Court and the Community Probation Service.

Despite the need to restructure, HAIP successfully kept its doors open. As the years progressed, HAIP expanded its initial three-staff team (Balzer 1999) to include ten part-time staff and about thirty to forty volunteers in 2002. (Today the Tuu Oho Mai agency is comprised of forty-five staff and one volunteer.) While it took a progressive approach, HAIP was ultimately failing to address the needs of its Māori clientele (Poata Watene, interview with Kanoelani R. Dodd, March 1, 2022).[1] Moreover, although it aimed to prevent the high number of Māori in prison, the mass incarceration of Māori remained consistent. Today Māori make up 15 percent of the general public, yet over 50 percent of incarcerated people (NZ Corrections 2022), a trend that has been consistent since the 1980s (Cunneen and Tauri 2019). Faced with the reality that HAIP was failing its Indigenous population, a decision was made to transition away from the Duluth Model to a *te ao Māori / kaupapa Māori* model; the website of Tuu Oho Mai Services (2021a) now states, "Our new vision is about building resilient whānau, and our purpose is about developing loving whānau so that they thrive."

TE AO MĀORI AND KAUPAPA MĀORI

The transition from the Western Duluth Model to *te ao Māori / kaupapa Māori* encompasses more than just a shift in ideology; it is a change in philosophy (Watene). *Kaupapa Māori* "is a movement of resistance and of revitalization, incorporating theories that are embedded within te ao Māori" (Berryman 2008, 3). *Te ao Māori* can be understood as the interconnectedness of us all, which is a recurring concept throughout Indigenous cultures worldwide. As suggested by Cunneen (2018), having such relations is vital in healing.

By instituting *te ao Māori / Kaupapa Māori,* Tuu Oho Mai ensured that Māori knowledge became pivotal in all decision-making. The centraliza-

---

1. All subsequent Watene citations refer to March 1, 2022, interview conducted by Kanoelani R. Dodd.

tion of Māori knowledge, as noted by Rameka and Paul-Burke (2015), is substantial because, historically, such knowledge was suppressed in favor of Western knowledge. This suppression not only perpetuated colonial ideologies of the superior/inferior dichotomy but, in the fullness of time, it failed Indigenous Peoples.

INSTITUTING AN INDIGENOUS-BASED APPROACH

With the appointment of Poata Watene as CEO, HAIP began its transition in 2020. Watene, a Māori practitioner, fluent *te reo Māori* speaker, and past senior executive within Prisons and Community of the New Zealand Department of Corrections for twelve years, credits the drive to reshape the agency to a fellow Māori who served as a cochair on the board of trustees that advises the agency. Through advocacy and education, it was determined that the current mainstream approach was fundamentally failing to provide culturally appropriate services (Watene). The challenge was then to determine how a historically mainstream agency with a Western model would successfully integrate *te ao Māori / kaupapa Māori* and philosophy into not just the agency but also into its workers, clientele, and the community. As outlined by Watene (2022), the answer was located in the rewriting of the programs, the shift in philosophy, and the importance of acknowledging Indigenous expertise as parallel to Western methods.

Important to the evolution of the organization was changing its name. Tuu Oho Mai, which holds several translations, including "to stand awakened," "self-realization," and "self-determination," was gifted to the agency from the local *hapū*, Ngāti Māhanga (Watene). As indicated by Watene (2022), the change in name captures the traditional interconnectedness shared among people, environment, and culture. One can hear and sense the difference between *Tuu Oho Mai* and the previous *Hamilton Abuse Intervention Project*; the former is in the language of the Māori and serves to connect people, whereas the latter lacked connection to Indigenous people, knowledge, and culture. In addition to the gifted name, the Ngāti Māhanga remain active in supporting Tuu Oho Mai. The integration between the local *hapū* and the agency attests to the cultural shift in Tuu Oho Mai, as such a partnership was not previously practiced or valued.

Fluent speakers, educators, and philosophers were needed for the rewriting of the agency's programs so that Western ideology and psychology did not dominate decisions about restorative pathway planning (Watene). Although psychological components remain in the programs, they are not central to the agency's operation. Applying Western knowledge to heal Indigenous Peoples is often ineffective, as spirituality, environment, and restorative justice practices may be omitted. As of 2022, Tuu Oho Mai has developed two distinctive paths: restorative and healing (Watene 2022). Both paths will be discussed in greater detail shortly.

As noted by Watene (2022), the Duluth Model did not contain *tikanga*—that is, Māori practices, protocols, and etiquette. Moreover, the fundamental goals of the program were not being met; therefore, a change in philosophy was required. Such changes included the structure of the programs, the interactions between clientele and staff, and the labels by which clientele were categorized. *Te ao Māori* (interconnectedness) is a central understanding for Māori, especially in times that require *manaakitanga* (support and generosity), when it can foster the conditions that encourage healing.

At Tuu Oho Mai, when people come together to share spaces, everyone is regarded with respect. Partaking in meals and songs is commonplace as cultural practices that bond people. Rather than utilizing the Western concept of a classroom, gathering spaces (referred to as *wānanga*) foster traditional ways of learning, as knowledge is shared among all in attendance (Watene 2022).

A final point in changes that the agency made includes how those who offend are perceived and thus labeled. Tannenbaum's (1999) labeling theory speaks extensively of the implications of labeling individuals, as the internalization of a label has lasting repercussions. At Tuu Oho Mai, individuals who offend are referred to as *rau puutohe* (eager blade). As explained by Watene (2022), *rau puutohe* are individuals who are not self-aware and who traditionally disregarded self-preservation in battle. It is in these Indigenous-based approaches that the restoration of *mana* begins. Restoring *mana* restores the interconnectedness Indigenous Peoples have always valued and relied on, and will continue to value and rely on into the future.

DISTINCTIVE PATHS: RESTORATIVE AND HEALING

Although labeled as distinctive, the restorative path and the healing path are interrelated. At Tuu Oho Mai, creating an environment where people feel connected back to their land is an ongoing process. For many Māori individuals, colonialism severed traditional ties to place and thus to each other; therefore, restoring those relations fosters a return to a more holistic lifestyle. For example, Watene (2022) notes the importance of healing the *wairua*, or spirit. *whatukura*, which is associated with male spirituality, corresponds with *māreikura*, which is female spirituality, and both were guardians of the upper heavenly realms. These two elements are equal, and in Dodd's understanding of *whatukura* and *māreikura*, they are likely equivalent to Kū and Hina in Hawaiian culture. These entities, when aligned, ensure balance.

By utilizing the *kaupapa* Māori construct and *te ao Māori* philosophy, the interrelatedness of male spirituality and perpetrating domestic violence becomes more visible. As stated by Watene (2022), the agency knows men are the primary aggressors in domestic violence, and the majority of the agency's male clients are Māori. Often with Māori offenders, there is a disconnect from traditional ways of being; therefore, spiritual healing is done on the *whatukura* line for the *rau puutohe*. *Whatukura*, as mentioned previously, concerns male spirituality and guardianship. Such healing, significantly, reminds Māori men that their ancestors were loving fathers, not just warriors (Watene 2022).

Spiritual healing for women who have experienced violence is equally important. As explained by Duran and Duran (1995, 29), exposure to violence intergenerationally may result in the manifestation of internalized and externalized violence. The repercussions of internalized violence include low self-worth, which can lead to substance abuse and suicide, whereas externalized violence against others manifests as domestic violence, child abuse, and even homicide (Nielsen and Robyn 2019). In restoring *māreikura*, the traditional values of Māori women as strong leaders, mothers, decision-makers, and educators begin to emerge.

Another aspect of healing self through healing spirituality occurs in learning genealogy and oratory. Learning where and from whom someone descends can indeed be empowering as they learn the histories of adversities, survival, resilience, and triumphs. In addition to learning one's lineage, oratory can also be used to connect people to place while providing cultural and personal wisdom. Such a story shared during Tuu Oho Mai programming speaks of Hinekauorohia, a Māori deity affiliated with sacred waters. As conveyed by Watene (2022), the reflective waters of Hinekauorohia remind people that they must be reflective in all that they do.

Details regarding specific programs offered at Tuu Oho Mai are discussed in the next section. This portion aims to elucidate some of the *kaupapa Māori* and *te ao Māori* philosophy, such as the importance of healing spirituality, knowing one's lineage, and creation stories. As stated by Watene (2022), "We have lost our way." Restoring Māori identity through processes like these contributes to the restoration of *mana*.

CURRENT OPERATIONS

In 2021, Tuu Oho Mai had about 4,500 clients, 68 percent of whom were Māori or other Oceanians. Tuu Oho Mai receives its clientele through mandated referrals or self-referrals. Mandated referrals come directly from the police, Ministry of Justice, Department of Corrections, and other collaborating agencies, and make up the bulk of all referrals. As noted by Watene (2022), mandating people to attend programs can be challenging, because the motivation to address behaviors and take responsibility is often absent. To combat these dilemmas, a highly motivated and skilled agency workforce that ensures effective, culturally responsive, and appropriate engagement is paramount (Watene).

Self-referrals come with their own set of challenges, as the government only pays Tuu Oho Mai to take 50 self-referrals annually. In 2020–21 alone, however, Tuu Oho Mai had 638 uncontracted self-referrals. As detailed by Watene (2022), that equates to 1,276 working hours for which Tuu Oho Mai was not paid. Rather than deny motivated individuals access to programs, the agency provides the services until it is out of the necessary resources. As asserted by Watene (2022), in the absence of providing those services, the status quo is perpetuated and these individuals are incarcerated.

Tuu Oho Mai receives funding from the police, the Ministry of Social Development, and Oranga Tamariki (Ministry for Children). Funders have different contracts with Tuu Oho Mai, such as providing for wrap-around services, social work, and violence crisis responses.

PROGRAMS

The transformation of Tuu Oho Mai is visible in the increase in its capacity. Ten years ago, HAIP delivered four programs; today, Tuu Oho Mai delivers sixteen simultaneously throughout the year. Those programs include *māreikura* (women's programs) and *whatukura* (men's programs).

Each program under *māreikura* explores a different theme. As explained by Watene (2022), one of those themes teaches of *mana wahine* (powerful women), with particular references to Māori women who have served as leaders and advocates throughout Aotearoa. The expectation is that being able to make connections with such people and places instills a sense of pride in the clients.

Overall objectives of *māreikura* include being able to recognize abusive behavior, exploring the causes and effects of living with violence, and understanding the impacts of this violence on family members, all the while prioritizing the safety of women and supporting them in rebuilding their lives (Tuu Oho Mai Services 2021b.) One *māreikura* program is aimed at women whose partners are attending *whatukura*. Here women learn how to ensure their own safety, how to measure any change in their partners, and what to expect while their partners are in programs (Tuu Oho Mai Services 2021b).

A second *māreikura* program, aimed at female domestic violence offenders, is a twenty-week group nonviolent education program that explores issues that allow abusive practices to happen. It provides participants with "a better understanding around the patterns of behavior that create situations of risk and harm to others and family" (Tuu Oho Mai Services 2021b). In addition to these programs, women who enter Tuu Oho Mai can receive aid with legal protection and social-economic support such as housing, employment, and income, in addition to having a *kaitiaki* (advocate) who serves to support and uplift their voices in whatever paths they decide to pursue, whether legal or not.

Whatukura is designed for men involved in domestic violence. Overarching objectives for the men's programs include examining belief systems and behaviors that lead to abuse; exploring risk management options and encouraging safe practices; expanding the definitions of violence and controlling behaviors; identifying and practicing noncontrolling alternatives; and lastly, discussing the effects of these behaviors on women, children, and men (Tuu Oho Mai Services 2021d).

Another service to note is the *whare* (shelter) Tuu Oho Mai provides to men issued with a police safety order (PSO). Police issue PSOs when, in response to incidents of family violence, the aggressor is required to leave the property (NZ Justice, n.d.). Providing shelter to men with PSOs has been a long-standing service of the agency; however, under its new operation model, Tuu Oho Mai now provides "a range of whanau services and programmes that include: pathways, court/systems advocacy, victim advocacy, offender accountability, safety planning, education programmes that focus on safety, whanau restoration and promoting non-violence for adults/whanau and tamariki" (Tuu Oho Mai Services 2021c). According to the Ministry of Justice (NZ Justice, n.d.), the prompt establishment of an effective service plan is essential for families, including those under a PSO, as violating any rules could ultimately result in probation or incarceration.

FOR MĀORI BY MĀORI

The integration of *kaupapa Māori* values and *te ao Māori* philosophy represents a significant shift, not just in ideology but in philosophy (Watene). Two standard requirements for Indigenous healing approaches, as outlined by Ward and Maruna (2007, 17), are that they are Indigenous controlled and are consistent with the principle of self-determination. Without these principles, the processes are likely to fail to address the needs of Indigenous Peoples.

Strong leadership and a team that believes in the importance of integrating Indigenous knowledge are ongoing requirements, in addition to the rewriting of programs, according to Watene (2022). Indigenous representation in any institution also likely aids in the success of the Indigenous participants, as they are able to see themselves in these role models. In the early years of HAIP, Māori made up 50 percent of the agency's personnel; today, they comprise about 90 percent of the workforce. As mentioned previously, the current clientele of Tuu Oho Mai is 68 percent Māori or other Oceanians, though that figure may likely increase with a recent rise in Māori personal partnerships with Samoans, Tongans, and Cook Islanders.

At Tuu Oho Mai, Watene (2022) notes, although the agency is fortunate to have its strong Māori workforce, not all of them grew up speaking *te reo Māori* or learning the traditional stories and customs. About a third of the workforce grew up within a traditional Māori setting, while the other two-thirds are currently on their own learning journeys. Because culturally appropriate services require significant investment, staff development and training at Tuu Oho Mai are ongoing. Teachings are often delivered by Māori cultural experts and include language and cultural lessons. Strengthening Māori identity, including for those working for the agency, has been fundamental in the agency's transformation (Watene 2022).

CHALLENGES

An ongoing challenge that Tuu Oho Mai faces is the lack of motivation clients often display when they are mandated to attend programs; however, as noted by Ross (2014), the threat of prison may be required to ensure some people are compliant with the aims of a program. Tuu Oho Mai no longer operates on a transactional level—that is, its interventions are no longer short term and lacking culturally significant engagement (Watene 2022). Instead, the agency's new mission is to provide effective, culturally responsive, and appropriate services for all clients, including those with mandated referrals.

Another challenge is clients who identify as other Pacific Islander yet lack connections to either Māori or their own culture. This requires staff to do research into their lineages. As noted by Watene (2022), though, it is common practice for Māori to reach out to partners in different regions to obtain cultural histories. Ultimately, the aim remains consistent: teach people from where and from whom they come, and in doing so, restore *mana* within self and community.

A final limitation of Tuu Oho Mai is the inability to take program participants into the outdoors. For Indigenous people, connection to the land is essential to being interconnected with life. The *ngāherehere* (bush, forest) and *moana* (ocean), as explained by Watene (2022), are significant to Māori; however, due to health and safety restrictions, taking supervised groups out is just not possible at the time of this writing. According to Watene (2022), the agency instead creates environments within Tuu Oho Mai where cultural normative practices such as eating food, singing, and *whakawhanaunga* (relational activities) are ever present.

FUTURE OF TUU OHO MAI

"We are all still on our journey," Watene (2022) reminded us. The transition of Tuu Oho Mai commenced only two years before this writing; therefore, evaluations regarding effectiveness will not occur until 2024 or 2025. It should be noted that when he was asked about evaluations measuring the success of the program after *te ao Māori / kaupapa Māori* integration, Watene (2022) countered with, "Who determines what success looks like?" As he asserts, the success of Indigenous healing approaches cannot be measured appropriately by Western standards that fail "to recognize the significance of spirituality and connectivity" (Watene).

CONCLUSION

Impacts of colonization, both deliberate and unintentional, remain observable in Aotearoa, with high rates of domestic violence among Māori individuals being just one. Traditionally, Māori women held diverse esteemed roles within society. As noted previously, the devaluing of Māori women by settler colonists was used to justify rape, exploitation, and violence (Nielsen and Robyn 2019). In addition to the subordination of Māori women, Māori men were stripped of their traditional roles. And, importantly, the dispossession of Māori people as a result of the Treaty of Waitangi contributed to the internalization and externalization of violence, which includes domestic violence (Nielsen and Robyn 2019).

In order to elevate Eurocentric notions of superiority, colonial ideologies deemed Indigenous Peoples, their knowledge, and their culture as inferior (Nielsen and Robyn 2019). Because of this, aspects of traditional life that historically connected Māori people together were suppressed. *Mana*, a concept that can be found throughout other areas of Oceania and served as a defining principle in Māori society in particular, transformed under Western influence. With the destruction of traditional relations, violence increased. In restoring one's *mana*, the balance of *hanau* (self), *whānau* (family), and community begins. Reclaiming one's identity, as stated by Rameka and Paul-Burke (2015, 265), "is a process of personal and cultural transformation that requires the unmasking of identities that are not one's own . . . identities inherited as a legacy of domination."

Tuu Oho Mai, formerly known as the Hamilton Abuse Intervention Project, has been serving Aotearoa for thirty years and has gone through a series of challenges that served to increase its resilience as a nonprofit agency run by and for Māori. Over the last three years, the agency has been engaged in a transition from the Western Duluth Model to the traditional *te ao Māori / kaupapa Māori* philosophy. Since the agency was failing to meet the needs of the majority of its clientele, Māori men, leadership determined that a restructuring of ideology and philosophy was needed. Reestablishing traditional visions of Indigenous life is the central ingredient of Indigenous healing practices (Ross 2014, 185). Through effective, culturally responsive, and appropriate engagement, Tuu Oho Mai aims to build resilience not only as an agency but within the *whānau* it serves. Because of this responsive and adaptive approach, Tuu Oho Mai will likely continue to serve Aotearoa well into the future.

REFERENCES

Balzer, Roma. 1999. "Hamilton Abuse Intervention Project: The Aotearoa Experience." In *Coordinating Community Response to Domestic Violence: Lessons from Duluth and Beyond*, edited by Melanie Shepard and Ellen Pence, 239–54. Sage Series on Violence Against Women. Thousand Oaks, CA: Sage Publications.

Busch, Ruth, and Neville Robertson. 1994. "'Ain't No Mountain High Enough (To Keep Me from Getting to You)': An Analysis of the Hamilton Abuse Intervention Pilot Project." In *Women, Male Violence and the Law*, edited by Julie Stubbs, 34–63. Sydney: Institute of Criminology.

Coates, Kenneth. 2004. *A Global History of Indigenous Peoples: Struggle and Survival*. New York: Palgrave Macmillan.

Cunneen, Chris. 2018. "Sentencing, Punishment and Indigenous People in Australia." SSRN Scholarly Paper. Rochester, NY: Social Science Research Network, April 30, 2018. https://papers.ssrn.com/abstract=321879.

Cunneen, Chris, and Juan Marcellus Tauri. 2019. "Indigenous Peoples, Criminology, and Criminal Justice." *Annual Review of Criminology* 2, no. 1: 359–81. https://doi.org/10.1146/annurev-criminol-011518-024630.

Duran, Eduardo, and Bonnie Duran. 1995. *Native American Postcolonial Psychology*. Albany: SUNY Press.

Durie, Mason. 1998. *Te Mana Te Kāwanatanga: The Politics of Māori Self-Determination*. Auckland: Oxford University Press.

Erai, Michelle. 2020. *Girl of New Zealand: Colonial Optics in Aotearoa*. Tucson: University of Arizona Press.

Fischer, Steven R. 2002. *A History of the Pacific Islands*. Basingstoke, UK: Palgrave Macmillan.

HAIP (Hamilton Abuse Intervention Project). 2001. "Early Detection of Children at Risk of Harm and Injury." Project proposal. Hamilton, NZ: Hamilton Abuse Intervention Project.

Hau'ofa, Epeli. 1994. "Our Sea of Islands." *Contemporary Pacific* 6, no. 1: 148–61. https://www.jstor.org/stable/23701593.

King, Michael, ed. 1992. *Te Ao Hurihuri: Aspects of Maoritanga*. Auckland: Reed.

Mezzadra, Sandro, and Brett Neilson. 2013. *Border as Method, or, the Multiplication of Labor*. Durham, NC: Duke University Press.

New Zealand Department of Corrections. 2022. "Prison Facts and Statistics—March 2022." https://www.corrections.govt.nz/resources/statistics/quarterly_prison_statistics/prison_stats_march_2022.

New Zealand Family Violence Clearinghouse. 2022. "Understanding the Impacts of COVID-19." https://nzfvc.org.nz/covid-19/FAQ-part-1.

Nielsen, Marianne O. and Samantha Brown. 2012. "Beyond Justice: What Makes an Indigenous Justice Organization?" *American Indian Culture and Research Journal* 36, no. 2: 47–73. https://doi.org/10.17953/aicr.36.2.m7441vm524166442.

Nielsen, Marianne O., and Linda M. Robyn. 2019. *Colonialism Is Crime*. New Brunswick, NJ: Rutgers University Press.

NZ Justice (New Zealand Ministry of Justice). n.d. "What Is a Police Safety Order?" Accessed March 11, 2023. https://www.justice.govt.nz/family/family-violence/whats-a-police-safety-order/.

NZ Justice (New Zealand Ministry of Justice). 2021. *New Zealand Crime and Victims Survey*. Wellington: Ministry of Justice. https://www.justice.govt.nz/assets/Documents/Publications/Cycle-3-Core-Report-20220224-v1.9.pdf.

Rameka, Lesley, and Kura Paul-Burke. 2015. "Re-Claiming Traditional Maori Ways of Knowing, Being, and Doing, to Re-Frame Our Realities and Transform Our Worlds." *Counterpoints* 500: 261–71. https://www.jstor.org/stable/i40222702.

Robertson, Neville R. 1999a. "Reforming Institutional Responses to Violence Against Women." PhD diss., University of Waikato.

Robertson, Neville R. 1999b. "Stopping Violence Programmes: Enhancing the Safety of Battered Women or Producing Better Educated Batterers?" *New Zealand Journal of Psychology* 28, no. 2: 68–78. https://www.psychology.org.nz /journal-archive/NZJP-Vol282-1999-1-Robertson.pdf.

Ross, Rupert. 2014. *Indigenous Healing: Exploring Traditional Paths.* Toronto: Penguin.

Salmond, Anne. 1997. *Between Worlds: Early Exchanges Between Maori and Europeans, 1773–1815.* Auckland: Viking.

Smith, Andrea. 2005. *Conquest: Sexual Violence and American Indian Genocide.* Cambridge, MA: South End Press.

Tannenbaum, F. 1999. "The Dramatization of Evil." In *Theories of Deviance,* edited by Stuart H. Traub and Craig B. Little, 380–84. Itasca, IL: F. E. Peacock Publishers.

Trask, Haunani-Kay. 1999. *From a Native Daughter: Colonialism and Sovereignty in Hawai'i.* Rev. ed. Honolulu: University of Hawai'i Press.

Tuu Oho Mai Services. 2021a. "Ko Wai Mātou (Our Story, Vision & Values)." https://www.tuuohomai.org.nz/about-tuuohomai/our-story-vision-values/.

Tuu Oho Mai Services. 2021b. "Maareikura: Women's Programmes." https://www .tuuohomai.org.nz/services/womens-programme/.

Tuu Oho Mai Services. 2021c. "Our Services." https://www.tuuohomai.org.nz /services/.

Tuu Oho Mai Services. 2021d. "Whatakura: Men's Programmes." https://www .tuuohomai.org.nz/services/mens-programme/.

UN Women. 2020. "COVID-19 and Ending Violence Against Women and Girls." https://www.unwomen.org/sites/default/files/Headquarters/Attachments /Sections/Library/Publications/2020/Issue-brief-COVID-19-and-ending -violence-against-women-and-girls-en.pdf.

Walker, Ranginui. 1990. *Ka Whawhai Tonu Matou: Struggle Without End.* Auckland: Penguin.

Ward, Tony, and Shadd Maruna. 2007. *Rehabilitation.* London: Routledge. https:// doi.org/10.4324/9780203962176.

CONCLUSION

KAREN JARRATT-SNIDER AND
MARIANNE O. NIELSEN

TOPICS WITHIN INDIGENOUS HEALTH and justice are so numerous and broad that they could fill multiple volumes. So many intersections exist—between health and environment, food, traditional medicines, water, spirituality, and so much more—that we could easily create a book dedicated to each of these Indigenous health and justice topics. Climate change overarches all these relationships and deserves an Indigenous justice book of its own. The multifaceted, tragic, and widespread impacts of COVID-19 in Indigenous Country could also fill a volume all by themselves. While many news stories about the pandemic in Indigenous Country focused on loss and tragedy, the resilience of Indigenous Peoples and their concern for non-Indigenous neighbors is also noteworthy. For example, as mentioned by Begay, Petillo, and Goldtooth in this volume, more than one Native nation in Oklahoma not only vaccinated their own citizens but also offered the vaccine to non-Indigenous persons (Mahoney 2021; Kemp 2022). Some Indigenous nations' testing, mitigation, and vaccination efforts became models for efficiency and effectiveness. In another example, the Chickasaw Nation created a drive-through facility for testing and vaccination that could accommodate 6,500 people per day, and both the Chickasaw and Cherokee Nations reported less than 100 active COVID cases at one point in July 2022 (Kemp 2022). With Cherokee being one of the largest Indigenous nations in the United States, less than 100 active cases offer evidence of the effectiveness of that nation's prevention and mitigation efforts (Kemp 2022). In this volume, the chapters from Begay, Petillo, and Goldtooth; Haskie; and Kunze and Camarillo offer further glimpses into some of the ways the pandemic affected Indigenous Country, and how Indigenous nations, communities, organizations, and leaders crafted responses to fill the gaps in the mostly inadequate, persistently underfunded, and culturally insensitive services provided to Indigenous Peoples by the federal governments of colonized countries (in the case of this volume, the United States, Canada, and Aotearoa / New Zealand). Federal governments are not living up to their obligations (called "trust obligations" in the United States) that are a matter of both domestic and international human rights law. However, in some countries, there have been strides forward; for example, in Australia, the Council for Aboriginal Reconciliation issued its final report in 2000 after over twenty years of work, and the Truth and Reconciliation Commission of Canada (Trudeau 2015) issued its final report in 2015. In both cases, the implementation of recommendations are as yet unclear. More recently in 2021, the federal government of Canada established Joyce's Principle that directly affects health-care services for Canada's Indigenous Peoples in that it "aims to guarantee all Indigenous Peoples the right of equitable access, without any discrimination, to all social and health services, as well as the right to enjoy the best possible physical, mental, emotional and spiritual health" (Department of Justice Canada 2021a).

Still, much remains to be done to achieve health equity for Indigenous Peoples. As Dietrich and Schroedel point out, the United States government spends less on Indigenous health care, proportionally, than on health care for the general population, and such underfunding has serious impacts on the health of Indigenous populations that use the Indian Health Service (IHS). Such negligence is implicated in significant health disparities, as the chapters by Dietrich and Schroedel and by Camplain et al. describe.

AMERICAN URBAN INDIANS AND HEALTH CARE

Health disparities are usually discussed in terms of Indian Country, but what is often forgotten is that about 87 percent of those who identify as American Indian or Alaska Native, alone or in combination, live away from Indigenous lands, with 70 percent living in urban areas where they are known to have "a frequency of poor health and limited health care options" (OMH 2022). The large urban Indigenous population is, in part, a function of settler colonialism and the attendant settler governments' policies. For example, U.S. federal termination and relocation policies (1945–60s) sent numerous Indigenous individuals and families to urban relocation centers in metropolitan areas such as Denver, Chicago, Minneapolis, Dallas, San Francisco, and other cities (Fixico 1986, 2000). Relocation, another iteration of assimilationist attempts, promised much to those who agreed to relocate. Often, though, the benefits actually provided to people who relocated were less than those promised, and they faced isolation from their communities, poverty, low-wage jobs, and discrimination (Fixico 1986, 2000; National Archives n.d.). Both termination and relocation officially ended with the ushering in of American Indian self-determination policy in the 1970s, but the Urban Indian Relocation Program already had created a large urban Indian population. Urban health services are just as necessary, and just as underfunded, as those available in Indian Country.

AMERICAN URBAN INDIAN CENTERS AND HEALTH CARE

More culturally sensitive, Indigenous-oriented programs are needed outside of Indian Country for the many Indigenous individuals who cannot come to Indian Country for help. U.S. urban Indian health-care centers such as the ones in Flagstaff and Salt Lake City, and thirty-nine clinics elsewhere, are an excellent start, but most are underfunded and located in old buildings with serious problems, as are their Indian Country counterparts (*Examining Federal Facilities in Indian Country* 2021). Urban Indian centers were established starting in the 1950s and '60s as a response to Indian relocation, and urban Indian populations' health needs became a significant contributing factor to the establishment of urban Indian clinics (Martin 2007). There are forty-one in existence as of 2022 (IHS, n.d.). Some manage to offer a wide array of programs, from behavioral health to family medicine, to care for those experiencing the long-term effects of COVID (see, e.g., the Tucson Indian Center 2022a). Some offer programs for known health issues, such as suicide prevention programs

(Tucson Indian Center 2022b) and youth programs that focus on the prevention of risky behavior among youth (Phoenix Indian Center 2019). Other urban Indian centers offer a wide range of programs and services, with limited health-care programs as part of their overall programming. Yet additional prevention and education programs are needed.

It is important to note that the IHS only provides services to members of federally recognized tribes, although there are many Indigenous Peoples that have either state recognition or no recognition at all from state or federal authorities (OMH 2022). Those within these groups must find health-care services elsewhere.

THE BREADTH OF INDIGENOUS HEALTH AND JUSTICE

Health organizations that serve Indigenous Peoples need to have a more holistic view of what health encompasses. As we see in this book, health and well-being encompass relationships with the land and water and all the beings that live in them, including people and the spirit world (see Thompson and Marek-Martinez; Dodd and Nielsen). From this point of view, a wide range of health-related issues originating in colonization become evident, including issues resulting from environmental degradation, climate change, pandemics, economic disadvantage, and racism. Important subpopulations of Indigenous people such as women and LGBTQ + individuals were special targets of colonial discrimination and threat and still are, as discussed in Nielsen and Jarratt-Snider (2023). Those harmed by internalized and externalized violence resulting from historical trauma also need additional resources since they are often left out of the research, policymaking, and funding. The acknowledgement of the impact of historical trauma and the incorporation of cultural resources as legitimate parts of health care are only beginning to be accepted outside of Indian Country, but they have been used extensively in some health-care facilities. For example, the Office of Native and Spiritual Medicine, part of the Tuba City Regional Health Care Corporation on the Navajo Nation, offers services include traditional counseling, diagnostic prayers, Diné cultural education, and "traditional Diné and Native American healing intervention" (TCRHCC 2019).

Indigenous Peoples have made important contributions to their own and others' health and well-being, as Begay, Petillo, and Goldtooth discuss. The story of the use of aspirin by Indigenous Peoples is fairly well known, but Indigenous Peoples of Turtle Island also invented syringes, pain relievers in addition to aspirin, oral birth control, sunscreen, baby bottles, mouth wash, and suppositories (Fisher 2020), and early vaccinations, sunscreen, and electrolyte rehydration (Advent Health 2022). They continue to contribute in a multitude of public health areas, including, among many others, climate justice, health, and well-being research; development of community health aide programs; development of new vaccines; becoming nurses, doctors, and other health-care professionals; and using Indigenous media to spread the word about prevention programs (CDC, n.d.). Moreover, some Indigenous nations within the United States are taking control of their own health-care systems, formerly under Bureau of Indian Affairs control. One such example, as discussed in Begay, Petillo, and Goldtooth, is the Cherokee Nation, which now operates two inpatient care facilities, including their own hospital (Cherokee Nation 2021).

In Australia, the National Aboriginal Community Controlled Health Organisation represents "145 Aboriginal Community Controlled Health Organisations (ACCHOs) that operate in over 300 clinics across Australia, delivering holistic, comprehensive and culturally competent primary health-care services. These ACCHOs are initiated and operated by local Aboriginal and Torres Strait Islander communities. The sector is the largest employer of Aboriginal and Torres Strait Islander people across Australia, with well over half of its 6,000 staff being Aboriginal and Torres Strait Islander" (NACCHO, n.d.). In Canada, federal and provincial governments fund health care for and by First Nations People, but there are issues. As the Department of Justice Canada (2021b) states, "A coordinated approach to address the health needs of First Nations, Inuit and Métis, and health-care delivery among all levels of government including Indigenous governments, remains an ongoing challenge. Improved clarity and a shared understanding of the role of various levels of government is needed, including for Métis, off-reserve First Nations and urban Inuit populations."

Not all Indigenous participation in health-care services has been intentional or willing. Traditional medicines, for example, have been stolen by corporations for decades through intellectual property theft. Citing data from Cultural Survival Canada, Grenier (1998, 16), writes, "The world market value of pharmaceuticals derived from plants used in traditional medicine had an estimated value of 43 billion United States dollars (USD) in 1985. Less than 0.001% of the profits has gone to the original holders of that knowledge." Imagine how much profit is being made by corporations thirty-eight years later and how little of it ends up in Indigenous communities, who could use it to develop more desperately needed health-care services and programs.

DE FACTO SOVEREIGNTY AND RESILIENCE

The authors in this volume point to the many areas of research that are still needed to assess health-care issues and the resilience that Indigenous Peoples and communities have shown in combating them. During the COVID pandemic, many Indigenous nations developed effective mechanisms for stopping the spread of the disease, including using cultural resources in communicating prevention strategies (see Begay, Petillo and Goldtooth; Haskie). For example, the Cherokee Nation asked its elders to record messages encouraging the population to get vaccinated. Success stories such as this need to be shared for the benefit of all Indigenous and non-Indigenous people, to help prepare for the next pandemic or other public health crisis. Strategies that help improve health care in general on a broader scale need to be shared. Every chapter in this volume describes a success story or suggests a successful strategy. More such publications are needed, and more research is needed that produces useful documents for Indigenous communities and organizations. Studies of Indigenous resilience itself are needed. Resilience is described as the foundation of survivance, but what goes into it? Can more successful strategies be described and shared?

More media-lobbying groups are needed to push back against discriminatory representations of Indigenous Peoples in the media. Organizations such as the National Congress of American Indians have been active in fighting the use of sports mascots, for instance, and they and other organizations need to be better funded, more visible, and treated more seriously by media organizations and information gatherers, especially in terms of such organizations' positive depictions of Indigenous resilience.

See the chapter by Kunze and Camarillo to get an understanding of the extent of the problem.

The many examples of de facto sovereignty operating in Indigenous communities need to be recognized and supported by federal government law, policy, and resources. There are legal barriers that prevent the provision of important services related to health care and well-being in Indigenous Country—the handling of violent crime, child neglect, and elder abuse are still not under the jurisdiction of tribal authorities, for example. These legal inadequacies are significant contributors to poor physical and mental well-being among Indigenous individuals. Healthcare services need to work in partnership with justice services, but this is extremely difficult under current federal law.

More universities, both Indigenous and non-Indigenous, need to partner with Indigenous communities and organizations to advance research and education for Indigenous community members and students. Northern Arizona University's Center for Health Equity Research, for example, has earned millions of dollars in grants with which to conduct health disparities research in partnership with Indigenous nations and communities in the Southwest (Center for Health Equity Research, n.d.).

As Indigenous Peoples, communities, and persons well know, the most effective solutions for Indigenous Country come from Indigenous people themselves. Indigenous nations and communities have been exercising de facto sovereignty and self-determination in order to find health-care solutions, as the Cherokee Nation and others have done, and to develop community-based programs and solutions, such as urban Indian health centers and other treatment programs. Indigenous Peoples, communities, and organizations continue to show their resilience and ingenuity in addressing the health needs of Indigenous people in the United States and worldwide.

REFERENCES

Advent Health. 2022. "8 Medical Contributions by Native Americans That Are Used Every Day." https://www.adventhealth.com/blog/8-medical-contributions-native-americans-are-used-every-day#.

CDC (Centers for Disease Control and Prevention). n.d. "Contributions to Public Health." Accessed July 2, 2023. https://www.cdc.gov/tribal/tribes-organizations-health/contributions/index.html.

Center for Health Equity Research. n.d. Accessed March 11, 2023. https://nau
.edu/cher/.

Cherokee Nation. 2021. "Health Services." Last updated August 26, 2021. https://
health.cherokee.org/health-center-and-hospital-locations/inpatient-care/.

Council for Aboriginal Reconciliation. 2000. *Final Report of the Council for Aboriginal Reconciliation to the Prime Mister and the Commonwealth Parliament.*
Canberra: Commonwealth of Australia, December 2000.http://www.austlii
.edu.au/au/other/IndigLRes/car/2000/16/index.htm.

Department of Justice Canada. 2021a. "Government of Canada Honours Joyce
Echaquan's Spirit and Legacy." Statement, September 28, 2021. https://www
.canada.ca/en/indigenous-services-canada/news/2021/09/government-of
-canada-honours-joyce-echaquans-spirit-and-legacy.html.

Department of Justice Canada. 2021b. "Indigenous Health Care in Canada."
https://www.sac-isc.gc.ca/eng/1626810177053/1626810219482.

*Examining Federal Facilities in Indian Country, Before the House Committee on Nat-
ural Resources, Subcommittee for Indigenous Peoples of the United States.* 2021.
"Testimony from Randy Grinnell, MPH on Examining Federal Facilities in
Indian Country Before House Committee on Natural Resources." June 17,
2021. https://www.hhs.gov/about/agencies/asl/testimony/2021/06/17/exam
ining-federal-facilities-indian-country.html.

Fisher, Nicole. 2020. "7 Native American Inventions That Revolutionized Medicine and Public Health." *Forbes*, November 29, 2020. https://www.forbes.com
/sites/nicolefisher/2020/11/29/7-native-american-inventions-that-revolution
ized-medicine-and-public-health/?sh=ff3cbf51e73b.

Fixico, Donald L. 1986. *Termination and Relocation: Federal Indian Policy, 1945–
1960.* Albuquerque: University of New Mexico Press.

Fixico, Donald L. 2000. *The Urban Indian Experience in America.* Albuquerque:
University of New Mexico Press.

Grenier, Louise. 1998. *Working with Indigenous Knowledge: A Guide for Researchers.*
Ottawa: International Development Research Centre.

IHS (Indian Health Service). n.d. "Urban Indian Organizations." https://www
.ihs.gov/urban/urban-indian-organizations/.

Kemp, Adam. 2022. "As COVID Swept the State, Native Communities in Oklahoma Raced to Preserve Culture." *Public Broadcasting Service News Hour*,
July 1, 2022. https://www.pbs.org/newshour/health/as-covid-swept-the-state
-native-communities-in-oklahoma-raced-to-preserve-culture.

Mahoney, Mike. 2021. "Native American Tribes in Oklahoma Look to Vaccinate
Friends and Neighbors." March 17, 2021. *KOAM News Now.* https://www
.koamnewsnow.com/news/coronavirus/native-american-tribes-in-oklahoma

-look-to-vaccinate-friends-and-neighbors/article_608de119-f588-520a-89b9
-f5f207863999.html.

Martin, Jessica. 2007. "Majority of American Indians Move Off-Reservation, but Their Cultural, Financial Resources Remain Behind." *Source*, April 12, 2007. St. Louis: Washington University at St. Louis. https://source.wustl.edu/2007 /04/majority-of-american-indians-move-off-reservations-but-their-cultural -financial-services-remain-behind/.

NACCHO (National Aboriginal Community Controlled Health Organisation). n.d. "Aboriginal Health in Aboriginal Hands." Accessed March 10, 2023. https:// www.naccho.org.au/#:~:text=Aboriginal%20health%20in%20Aboriginal%20 hands&text.

National Archives. n.d. "American Indian Urban Relocation." Accessed March 11, 2023. https://www.archives.gov/education/lessons/indian-relocation.html.

Nielsen, Marianne O., and Karen Jarratt-Snider, eds. 2023. *Indigenous Justice and Gender*. Tucson: University of Arizona Press.

OMH (Office of Minority Health). 2022 "Profile: American Indian/Alaska Native." U.S. Department of Health and Human Services. https://minorityhealth .hhs.gov/omh/browse.aspx?lvl=3&lvlid=62.

Phoenix Indian Center. 2019. "Prevention Services." https://phxindcenter.org /prevention-services/.

TCRHCC (Tuba City Regional Health Care Corporation). 2019. "Office of Native and Spiritual Medicine." https://www.tchealth.org/onsm/.

Trudeau, Justin. 2015. "Final Report of the Truth and Reconciliation Commission of Canada." Press release. December 15, 2015. https://pm.gc.ca/en/news/back grounders/2015/12/15/final-report-truth-and-reconciliation-commission -canada.

Tucson Indian Center. 2022a. "Health Services Department." https://www.ticenter .org/health-services-department/#:~:text=COVID%2D19%20Chronic%20 Care%20%E2%80%93%20The,of%20infection%20or%20re%2Dinfection.

Tucson Indian Center. 2022b. "Suicide Prevention." https://www.ticenter.org/sui cide-prevention/.

CONTRIBUTORS

Julie Baldwin (citizen of Cherokee Nation of Oklahoma) is a Regents' Professor in the Department of Health Sciences, executive director of the Center for Health Equity Research, and NARBHA vice-president for NAU Health at Northern Arizona University (NAU). She earned her doctorate in behavioral sciences and health education from the Johns Hopkins Bloomberg School of Public Health. From 1994 to 2004, she served as a tenured faculty member at NAU. She joined the faculty at the University of South Florida College of Public Health in the Department of Community and Family Health in 2005. She returned to NAU in July 2015. Dr. Baldwin's research over the years has focused on both infectious and chronic disease prevention. She has had a consistent program of applied research addressing HIV/AIDS and substance abuse prevention in youth, with a special emphasis on working with American Indian youth and their families.

Manley A. Begay Jr. (Navajo) is a tenured professor in the Department of Applied Indigenous Studies and Department of Politics and International Affairs at the College of Social and Behavioral Sciences at Northern Arizona University (NAU) in Flagstaff. Professor Begay is also an affiliate faculty member of the W. A. Franke College of Business at NAU, as well as the director of the Tribal Leadership Initiative in the Office of Native American Initiatives at NAU. His major specialization lies at the heart of issues pertaining to Indigenous nation building, sovereignty, governance, culture, leadership, education, economic development, and Navajo philosophy. Further, his work includes executive education sessions and research, with and relevant to First Nations and organizations in Canada, Native nations and organizations in the United States, and Indigenous organizations elsewhere.

Earlene Camarillo is an associate professor in the Department of Politics, Policy, and Administration at Western Oregon University. Her expertise includes the American political system, health policy, and public administration. Her research centers on the interactions of health, policy, and public organizations. Dr. Camarillo's current projects include an investigation into the impact of the coronavirus on local health departments and a project examining the role of the media in COVID-19 response for Native American communities.

Carolyn (Carly) Camplain (Comanche) is an assistant professor of Indigenous health law and policy in the Department of Community and Population Health and a researcher with the Institute for Indigenous Studies at Lehigh University in Bethlehem, Pennsylvania. Her research interests are in health and health-care access of Indigenous people in jails and prisons, including those incarcerated in tribal jails. She wants to bridge the gap between law and science to address systemic racism and to advocate for health equity. Dr. Camplain is licensed to practice law in the state of New Mexico.

Ricky Camplain (Comanche) is an assistant professor in the Department of Epidemiology and Biostatistics at the Indiana University School of Public Health. Her research combines epidemiologic methods and community-based participatory research to determine how the cultural, social, structural, and political environments in correctional facilities impact health among people incarcerated, particularly those at the intersection of being Indigenous and incarcerated.

Carmenlita Chief, MPH, is Diné (Navajo) from the Navajo Nation community of Tó Dínéeshzhee'. She is Kinłichii'nii (Red House Clan) and born for Lok'aa' Dine'é (Reed People). Her maternal grandfathers are Honágháahnii (One Who Walks Around Clan) and her paternal grandfathers are Yé'ii Dine'é Tachii'nii (Giant People of the Red Running into the Water Clan). Carmenlita is a senior research coordinator for the Center for Health Equity Research at Northern Arizona University, and she has published numerous scientific articles in the areas of health equity, community-based participatory research, Indigenous health and cultural health frameworks, and cancer prevention. Outside of academia, Carmenlita is involved in local community initiatives advocating for Indigenous wellness, connectedness, and recognition in the border town of Flagstaff, Arizona.

Joseph Dietrich works closely on political engagement, voter disenfranchisement, and voting by mail in the Native American community. Currently, he is conducting a study on access to voting among minority populations, in which he is co-developing a tool to measure voting equity. He has over twenty years of research experience in polling and survey research, voting and political behavior, elite interviews, race and ethnic politics, and the intersection of politics, policy, and education. He holds a PhD in social and comparative analysis from the University of Pittsburgh and a PhD in political science from Claremont Graduate University. He currently teaches politics and public policy at the California State Polytechnic University, Pomona.

Kanoelani R. Dodd is a Kanaka Maoli (Native Hawaiian) from Waikapū, Maui. Ms. Dodd has a master's degree in applied criminology from Northern Arizona University. Upon receiving her bachelor of arts in administration of justice from the University of Hawai'i at Hilo, Ms. Dodd worked as a probation officer for the State of Hawai'i. Ms. Dodd is interested in Indigenous justice in a variety of areas, including settler colonialism, the criminal justice system, tourism, and resiliency. Ms. Dodd aims to provide an Indigenous voice in both academia and the criminal justice system.

Carol Goldtooth (Navajo) is the outreach program coordinator and community health educator for the Partnership for Native American Cancer Prevention (NACP) at Northern Arizona University. She works to bridge gaps by providing technical assistance and supporting tribal capacity building for cancer education, programming, and research with

NACP. She earned her master of public health degree from the University of Arizona. Her professional focus has been on culturally appropriate, community-based, participatory approaches to addressing health disparities and chronic disease like diabetes; heart disease prevention and management; cancer prevention and education; child and family health; and elucidating connections between health and Indigenous nation building.

Miranda Jensen Haskie (Diné), PhD, is a professor of sociology in the School of Business and Social Science at Diné College in Tsaile, Navajo Nation, Arizona. Her publications include *Future of Navajo Education*, co-edited with Barbara Mink and Kathy Tiner (Fielding University Press, 2021); "Hozho Nahasdlii—Finding Harmony in the Long Shadow of Colonialism: Two Perspectives on Teaching Anti-Racism at a Tribal College" with Bradley Shreve, in K. Haltinner's *Teaching Race in Contemporary America* (2013); and "Teaching Sociology at a Tribal College: Navajo Philosophy as a Pedagogy" in the *American Sociologist* (2013).

Lomayumtewa K. Ishii (Hopi) is a 2016 Rollin and Mary Ella King Native Artist Fellow in the School for Advanced Research in Santa Fe, New Mexico. After completing his fellowship, Mr. Ishii worked with the HeArt Box Gallery in Flagstaff, Arizona, on an exhibition called *Sinom* ("the People" in Hopi). The exhibition focused on Mr. Ishii's traditional knowledge in a series of twelve works, which were also published in the *Phoenix Home & Garden* August 2020 issue. His work also has been featured in the *Northern Arizona Mountain Living* August 2020 issue and in the *Arizona Daily Sun* September 2015 issue.

Karen Jarratt-Snider (Choctaw descent) is a professor in the Department of Applied Indigenous Studies at Northern Arizona University. Her expertise is in the areas of Indigenous environmental justice, management, and policy; federal Indian policy, tribal administration, sustainable economic development, and tribal environmental management—all of which coalesce around the overall topic of Indigenous sovereignty and self-determination. She has over fifteen years of experience working with tribal nations' projects in applied, community-based research.

Stefanie Kunze holds a PhD in political science and is an assistant professor in the Department of Sociology at Northern Arizona University. Dr. Kunze specializes in perpetrators of genocide and ethnocide, Native American experiences with settler colonialism and assimilation, and related political, societal, and social challenges. Her current work is focused on perpetrators of ethnocide in Native America, comparative approaches to the United States' boarding school legacy, and policy responses to pandemic-related needs in tribal communities.

Ora V. Marek-Martinez's (Navajo, Nez Perce, and Hopi) work includes ensuring the success of Northern Arizona University (NAU) Indigenous students through Indigenized programming and services. Dr. Marek-Martinez's research as an Anthropology Department assistant professor includes Indigenous archaeology, research and approaches that utilize ancestral knowledge, decolonizing and Indigenizing methodologies, and storytelling in the creation of archaeological knowledge to reaffirm Indigenous connections to land. Dr. Marek-Martinez is a founding member of the Indigenous Archaeology Collective and is associate vice president for Native American Initiatives at NAU.

Marianne O. Nielsen is a professor emerita in the Department of Criminology and Criminal Justice at Northern Arizona University. She is the co-author of *Colonialism Is Crime* (2019) with Linda M. Robyn and *Finding Right Relations: Quakers, Native Americans, and Settler Colonialism* with Barbara M. Heather (2022). She is the co-editor with Robert A. Silverman of *Aboriginal Peoples and Canadian Criminal Justice* (1992), *Native Americans, Crime, and Criminal Justice* (1996), and *Criminal Justice in Native America* (2009); with James W. Zion of *Navajo Peacemaking: Living Traditional Justice* (2005); and with Karen Jarratt-Snider of *Crime and Social Justice in Indian Country* (2018), *Traditional, National, and International Law and Indigenous Communities* (2020), *Indigenous Environmental Justice* (2020), and *Indigenous Justice and Gender* (2023).

Leola Tsinnajinnie Paquin (Diné/Filipina and accepted into Santa Ana Pueblo), PhD, is an assistant professor of Native American studies at the University of New Mexico (UNM). Her research and service activities focus on Indigenous educational sovereignty. She is an associated faculty member with UNM's Institute for American Indian Education, has co-chaired the UNM Diversity Council Curriculum Subcommittee, been a UNM Academic Affairs General Education Faculty Fellow on Race and Social Justice, and is a former council president of the national American Indian Studies Association. Most recently, she has been focusing on Indigenous education initiatives with school districts and colleges in New Mexico.

April D. J. Petillo is an assistant professor of public sociology at Northern Arizona University, concentrating on gender, sexuality, race/ethnicity, political status, and culture. Community social justice inspires April's interdisciplinary, comparative analysis of safety and protection through the experiences of Indigenous, Black, and otherwise marginalized peoples. April's primary projects highlight legally encoded ethnic, racial, gendered, and sexualized politics as well as multifaceted coalition and community building.

Jean Reith Schroedel is the emerita Thornton Bradshaw Professor of Politics and Policy at Claremont Graduate University. She has written or co-edited six books, including *Is the Fetus a Person? A Comparison of Policies Across the Fifty States*, which was given APSA's Victoria Schuck Book Award, as well as more than fifty scholarly articles. In 2017, she was awarded the Claremont Colleges Diversity in Teaching Award. Her recent research has focused on voting rights issues affecting Native Americans. Dr. Schroedel was an expert witness in the *Wandering Medicine v. McCulloch* and *Yazzie v. Hobbs* cases and did research that was used in the *Poor Bear v. Jackson County* and *Sanchez v. Cegavske* cases. Her most recent book, *Voting in Indian Country: The View from the Trenches* (2020), is an outgrowth of this research.

Nicolette I. Teufel-Shone is a professor in the Department of Health Sciences and the associate director of the Center for Health Equity Research at Northern Arizona University in Flagstaff. As a public health scholar, she collaborates with Native nations to support the development of effective culturally anchored community health programs. With Indigenous graduate students and/or community partners, she has co-authored more than sixty peer-reviewed articles addressing Indigenous health and promising practices. Her work strives to achieve health equity through chronic disease prevention and promotion of healthy lifestyles.

Kerry F. Thompson, PhD, is a citizen and resident of the Navajo Nation. She is an Indigenous archaeologist whose research interests focus on the inclusion of Indigenous perspectives and paradigms in archaeology, tribal cultural resource management, Diné identity, and Native American representation. The foundation of Dr. Thompson's career in archaeology is the southwestern United States, primarily the Colorado Plateau. She is currently an associate professor and department chair in anthropology at Northern Arizona University.

INDEX